ROYAL HISTORICAL SOCIETY

STUDIES IN HISTORY

New Series

MEDICAL CHARITIES, MEDICAL POLITICS

MEDICAL CHARITIES, MEDICAL POLITICS

THE IRISH DISPENSARY SYSTEM AND THE POOR LAW, 1836–1872

Ronald D. Cassell

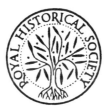

THE ROYAL HISTORICAL SOCIETY

THE BOYDELL PRESS

First published 1997

A Royal Historical Society publication
Published by The Boydell Press
an imprint of Boydell & Brewer Ltd
PO Box 9   Woodbridge   Suffolk IP12 3DF   UK
and of Boydell & Brewer Inc.
PO Box 41026   Rochester   NY 14604–4126   USA

ISBN 0 86193 228 5

ISSN 0269–2244

A catalogue record for this book is available
from the British Library

Library of Congress Cataloging-in-Publication Data
Cassell, Ronald Drake, 1934–
    Medical charities, medical politics : the Irish dispensary system and the Poor
Law, 1836–1872 / R.D. Cassell.
        p. cm. – (Royal Historical Society studies in history. New series,
ISSN 0269–2244)
    Includes bibliographical references and index.
    ISBN 0–86193–228–5 (hardback : alk. paper)
    1. Poor – Medical care – Ireland – History – 19th century. 2. Poor – Medical
care – Law and legislation – Ireland. 3. Poor – Medical care – Government policy
– Ireland – History – 19th century. 4. Charities, Medical – Ireland – History –
19th century. I. Royal Historical Society (Great Britain) II. Title. III. Series.
    [DNLM: 1. Health Services – history – Ireland. 2. Poverty – history –
Ireland. 3. Health Services – Ireland – legislation. 4. Health Policy – history –
Ireland. 5. Charities – history – Ireland. WA 11 GI6 C3ma 1997]
RA412.5.I7C37 1997
362.1'09415'09034 – dc21
DNLM/DLC
for Library of Congress   97–3751

This publication is printed on acid-free paper

Printed in Great Britain by
St Edmundsbury Press Ltd, Bury St Edmunds, Suffolk

Contents

Abbreviations

BL   British Library
DMP   *Dublin Medical Press*
DNB   *Dictionary of National Biography*
IPLC   Irish Poor Law Commission
PRO   Public Record Office

Parliamentary papers

Bromley-Stephenson report	Madox Bromley and W. H. Stephenson, *Report on the poor law department (Ireland) to the Lord's commissioners of Her Majesty's Treasury*, PRO, Treasury papers, T. 1/5906
Lambert report	*Twentieth and fifteenth annual report*, appendix C, iv (HC 1867, xxxiv)
Lord's committee (1846)	*Report by the Lords' select committee appointed to inquire into the operation of the 1 & 2 Vict. c. 56, and the other laws relating to the relief of the destitute poor in Ireland; and also to inquire into the operation of the medical charities in Ireland* (HC 1846, xi)
Poor Law Commission report (1841)	*Report of the poor law commissioners on the medical charities (Ireland)* (HC 1841, xi)
Royal Commission report	Report of the Royal Commission on the poor laws and relief of distress, appendix ii, *Poor law dispensary medical relief in Ireland* (HC 1910, i)
Select committee (1830)	*Report of the select committee of the House of Commons on the state of the poor in Ireland* (HC 1830, vii)
Select committee (1843)	*Report of the select committee of the House of Commons on the Irish medical charities* (HC 1843, x)
Whately report (1835)	*First report of the commissioners inquiring into the condition of the poor in Ireland, Appendix B* (HC 1835, xxxii)

Preface

Ruth Barrington has observed that by 1970 access to medical care had become a 'social right of citizenship' in Ireland.[1] That such a historically poor and politically fractured country should have managed to establish such a generous system of state medicine is a noteworthy achievement. While largely inspired by various welfare state models which had been developed in post World War II Europe, especially that of Britain, such a system also had deep roots in Ireland's past. This study examines some of them.

It began as an effort to explore in detail Oliver MacDonagh's assertion that in the first half of the nineteenth century Ireland had, insofar as policy and administrative structure were concerned, 'one of the most advanced health services in Europe . . . [and that it was] . . . to a large degree state supported, uniform and centralised'.[2] In the course of preliminary reading I discovered the Medical Charities Act of 1851, what the Irish customarily referred to as the Dispensary Act because it placed the dispensaries under the Irish Poor Law Commission. It soon became clear that it was of central importance to the whole story and I shifted the focus of my research to explain its origins and the effect it had upon medical relief and epidemic control in Ireland up to the conversion of the Irish Poor Law Commission into the Local Government Board in 1872. Thus the work came to cover both the pre-famine medical charities and the reorganised poor law system which largely supplanted them at mid-century.

In addition, the book came to devote far more attention to medical politics than I could have anticipated in the beginning. The angry quarrels of the doctors over standards of education and professional status, both with laymen and with each other, were intertwined with the relationship of the profession to the state and to various forms of state-subsidised medical relief. In particular, the relationship of the medical men with the poor law authority was a constant feature of the period. I found I could not understand the latter without placing it within the larger context of British medical politics in general. Consequently, the book devotes considerable space to the detailed examination of efforts to pass various medical charities measures between the 1830s and the 1860s. Some readers may find the blow-by-blow discussion of what were mostly failed attempts at reform both tedious and not very useful; those I invite to skip ahead to sections they find more interesting. But, for a number of reasons, it has seemed worthwhile to devote some space to this

---

[1] Ruth Barrington, *Health, medicine and politics in Ireland 1900–1970*, Dublin 1987, 1.
[2] Oliver MacDonagh, *Ireland*, Englewood Cliffs, NJ 1968, 27.

topic. It is true that there are a number of accounts of the struggle for medical reform in England and of the battles between the profession and the poor law authority, though even these are now rather dated, but there is no treatment of the Irish efforts in this area. In addition, the most recent examination of the evolution of Irish health policy, Barrington's excellent study, is focused on the twentieth century and provides only a perfunctory introduction to nineteenth-century developments paying little attention to the medical politics of the Victorian era. They require close examination to gain an adequate understanding of the issues involved, the difficulties against which the various parties struggled, and, therefore, the compromised and incomplete character of the legislation which finally reached the books. Moreover, only detailed treatment can recapture the particular sense of the times and the key personalities. I concluded that understanding the politics of medical charities reform was the only way to grasp the context within which the Medical Charities Act emerged, a context which largely defined both the limits and the strengths of state medicine in Ireland in this period.

Finally, I was led to think that the Irish way of administering poor law medical relief and epidemic control under the Medical Charities Act had influenced reform in England in the late 1860s and early 1870s. The study therefore concludes with an examination of the debate over public health and poor law medical charity reform in England in those decades, specifically with the Metropolitan Poor Act of 1867 and the formation of the English Local Government Board in 1871, and the important quarrel between John Lambert and John Simon over the nature of state medicine in England in the 1870s.[3] It seemed a long way from the original focus of the project and yet an unavoidable implication which cried out to be explored and integrated into the whole work. In the end, then, the book came to cover a good deal more ground than originally intended. It fails to fit neatly into any of the conventional national or topical categories: it necessarily involves Ireland and England, politics and administration, the poor law, medicine and public health.

I have incurred many debts in the years it has taken to complete this book. Most prominent is that owed to Dick Soloway, now chairman of the Department of History, University of North Carolina at Chapel Hill, who encouraged my interest in Irish administration, refused to accommodate a tendency toward rambling incoherence in early drafts, and provided cheerful support in moments of despair or panic. I recall going to him in such a state shortly before departing for Ireland to do the archival research. I had been misled by the mention of poor law records among the chief secretary's papers in the Irish State Paper Office into thinking that the full run of poor law authority

---

[3] The standard treatments of this important episode are found in Royston Lambert, *Sir John Simon 1816–1904 and English social administration*, London 1963, 501–77, and Jeanne L. Brand, *Doctors and the state: the British medical profession and government action in public health, 1870–1912*, Baltimore 1965, 7–31. See also the account of the medical officer himself: Sir John Simon, *English sanitary institutions*, 2nd edn, London 1897, 323–92.

records were housed there. An inquiry to the deputy keeper had revealed that in fact the Poor Law Commission and Local Government Board records had been destroyed in the IRA raid on the Customs House in 1921. I thought the project doomed. Dick refused to be impressed. 'They all say that', he muttered, referring apparently to archivists in general, 'Go on over and dig up what you can. There's more there than they think.' His aggressive confidence was vindicated by the result. In fact, the material in the files of the chief secretary's office, though uneven and far from complete, turned out to be an important and unappreciated resource for Irish poor law history. Other members of the UNC history department were helpful as well: Gillian Cell, now Provost at William and Mary College, and Michael McVaugh brought their special expertise to bear upon the project, to its great profit; Steven Baxter generously encouraged what I am sure appeared to him to be an unpromising and unconventional student; the late Jim Godfrey smoothed my path in many ways, not least through his incomparable experience with the university administration; and John Nelson provided more moral support than he knows. I am grateful to them all.

Others provided crucial assistance at various stages of the project also. Richard Bardolph, head of the Department of History at the University of North Carolina at Greensboro for many years, made my 1973 research leave possible, bending a few rules in the process. Colleagues Ann Pottinger Saab and Bill Link read the entire manuscript and made important suggestions for its improvement. John Eyler of the University of Minnesota and Martin Daunton of University College London, generously did the same and, in addition, provided encouragement at a critical moment on the road toward publication. Bob Calhoon, as he has done for nearly thirty years, gave steady support and advice. Whatever errors may remain are entirely my own.

A Summer Research Fellowship from the UNCG Research Fund made possible archival work in London and Salisbury in 1978. A subsequent research leave in 1987 permitted valuable rewriting and revision.

No work of this sort can be done without the inestimable aid of the staffs of numerous archives and libraries. I am especially indebted to the personnel of the State Paper Office in Dublin and to the then deputy keeper, Mr MacGiolla Choille, whose kindly interest in the project of an inexperienced historian helped run to earth many an elusive file. Mrs Brigid Dolan, librarian of the Royal Irish Academy, was also especially helpful as were the librarians, archivists and staffs of the National Library of Ireland, the library of Trinity College, Dublin, the Cork County Archives, Cork, the libraries of the Royal College of Physicians and the Royal College of Surgeons, Dublin, the Public Record Office at Chancery Lane and Kew, the British Library, the University College Library, London, the Ministry of Health Library in the Department of Health and Social Security, London, the Bodleian Library, Oxford, the Wiltshire Record Office, Salisbury, and the library of the Welcome Institute for the History of Medicine, London. The staffs and resources of the libraries at the University of North Carolina at Chapel Hill and Duke University and the libraries of medicine at those two universities and the History of Medicine Library of the National Library of Medicine in Bethesda, Maryland, were vitally important as well. I owe special thanks to the staff of the Walter Clinton Jackson Library of the University of North Carolina at Greensboro, and especially to the interlibrary loan librarians who have promptly and uncomplainingly met my every request.

In this electronic age other technical support has become necessary. I have been well served by the Academic Computing Center at UNCG, headed by Marlene Pratto, which has frequently dragged me kicking and screaming from one word processing upgrade to another, refusing to be defeated by someone as resistant to technology as ageing historians are prone to be. Diane Case Schabinger and Judy Martin guided me over many a technical barrier and this book would not be what it is without their patience and expertise.

Chapter iii of this book is based substantially on an article published in *Medical History* xxiv (1990), and I am grateful to the editors of that journal and to the Wellcome Institute for permission to reproduce it here.

I also wish to thank the Royal Historical Society for its interest in this book and particularly Christine Linehan who has been a skilful and supportive trans-Atlantic editor.

Finally, I owe most to Barbara who made it all possible.

Ronald D. Cassell
January 1997

1

The Irish Medical Charities
Before 1851

The Irish medical charities appeared in the eighteenth and nineteenth centuries as part of a larger movement which saw the establishment of hospitals and other medical facilities throughout the British Isles.[1] In its broadest sense the term came to embrace a wide variety of institutions ranging from simple one-room dispensaries to large hospitals, and from all-purpose facilities to those specialising in the treatment of specific diseases and conditions, such as incurables, fever, venereal disease, or the insane. Though differing widely in size, purpose and administrative organisation, all were considered to be medical charities so long as their funds were largely or wholly contributed by private donors or were drawn from endowments or government subsidy, or their medical personnel served without remuneration, or their treatment and medicines were dispensed gratuitously.

However, this study uses the term somewhat more narrowly. In Ireland by the 1830s and 1840s the medical charities came to be associated primarily with those institutions that were the focus of a movement to improve and expand the basic medical care provided to the poor across the entire country. By that time the voluntary hospitals in Dublin and Belfast were already well provided for by endowments and state subsidies, and the mentally ill were served by a group of state asylums which had been built, rather lavishly some thought, under the provisions of the Asylums Act of 1817 and subsequent amending legislation.[2] What remained, the vast bulk of Irish medical institutions, consisted of the country infirmaries, the fever hospitals and the dispensaries. As reformers pressed for medical charities legislation from 1835 onward it was these institutions with which they were concerned.

In the eighteenth and early nineteenth centuries Ireland remained an overwhelmingly rural and agricultural country which, none the less, was

[1] The following works provide a valuable introduction to the hospital movement and the emergence of the humanitarian impulse in eighteenth- and nineteenth-century England: John Woodward, *To do the sick no harm: a study of the British voluntary hospital system to 1875*, London–Boston 1974; Brian Abel-Smith, *The hospitals 1800–1948: a study in social administration in England and Wales*, Cambridge, Mass. 1964; David Owen, *English philanthropy 1660–1960*, Cambridge, Mass. 1964; and Keith Thomas, *Religion and the decline of magic*, New York 1971.
[2] Mark Finnane, *Insanity and the insane in post-famine Ireland*, London 1981, ch. i.

experiencing strong commercial and industrial development which in turn was producing prosperous urban pockets, largely in Ulster and Leinster, amid the traditional agrarian poverty.[3] Partly as a consequence of these changing economic and social circumstances, substantial and sustained growth in population set in from roughly the middle of the eighteenth century: about 2 million in 1767, it more than doubled by 1801 and swelled to over 8.5 million by 1845. Complicating the picture further was the dependence of a large portion of the agricultural labourer population upon a single crop, potatoes, a food which maintained health and vigour if available in sufficient quantity but the failure of which periodically created terrible subsistence crises culminating in the catastrophe of 1845–9. Epidemics invariably accompanied these disasters and endangered the entire community.[4]

The need for a system of medical charity which would be national in scope and geared to provide care for that large element of the population which could not afford to pay for it, was, many came to think, increasingly obvious under these conditions. In England, though the potential for subsistence crises was not as great, a powerful humanitarian movement was generating a growing charitable commitment to building and funding voluntary hospitals and dispensaries. However, the emerging English models, based as they were upon abundant charitable resources, were not applicable to many regions in Ireland where the gentry and the middle classes were comparatively small and poor. The factor which precipitated the creation of the first country-wide set of medical charities, the county infirmaries, was related to this absence of financial resources in the countryside. Outside Dublin and the larger towns the families that could afford professional care were spread so thinly on the ground that it made no financial or professional sense for physicians or surgeons to establish practices.[5] Furthermore, medical education was in its infancy in Ireland and few able young men were entering the profession. In 1765 the Irish parliament sought to remedy both these conditions by passing the Infirmaries Act (5 & 6 Geo. III, c. 20) which permitted the creation of an infirmary in every county except Dublin and Waterford, both of which already possessed such facilities. Though permissive rather than mandatory, a common feature of much eighteenth- and early nineteenth-century social legislation, the Infirmaries Act proved a considerable success and established

3 Much interesting and detailed work has recently been done on demographic and economic aspects of this period. The most useful summaries are found in Roy Foster, *Modern Ireland 1600–1972*, London 1989, 109–205, 217–19, 319–20, and Cormac O Grada, 'Poverty, population, and agriculture, 1801–45', in W. E. Vaughn (ed.), *Ireland under the Union, I: 1801–70*, Oxford 1989, 108–28.

4 There were fourteen partial or complete potato failures between 1816 and 1842: Foster, *Modern Ireland*, 320.

5 Medicus, *Observations and suggestions on the medical charities of Ireland*, Dublin 1851, 1–2.

a general administrative and funding model from which other forms of medical charity could be derived.[6]

The act provided that an infirmary could be established in each county under the supervision of a governing corporation, which was to be composed of certain ranking dignitaries such as the primate and lord chancellor of Ireland, the bishop of the diocese in which the infirmary was situated, and other local notables, as well as persons who contributed to its revenues. These latter, who invariably constituted the vast majority of the corporation's membership, were of two types: life members who had donated twenty guineas or more, and annual subscribers of at least three guineas.[7]

Each corporation was responsible for managing the finances of its infirmary and defining policy on admissions, selecting the surgeon and other personnel, maintaining the buildings etc. Such duties were rarely demanding. While some corporations met monthly and insisted on making decisions themselves, most delegated such matters to a smaller subcommittee or to the surgeon himself. If corporate obligations were usually light the privileges of membership came to be highly regarded. They assumed two forms: the right to recommend patients for treatment and the right to vote for the infirmary surgeon.

Admission to an infirmary required residency in the county and the acquisition of a ticket. The latter could only be obtained from members of the corporation or from the surgeon himself who frequently had full authority to admit whomsoever he thought appropriate. In theory the objects of relief were to be the worthy poor who would be given tickets upon application to a member of the corporation which they would then present at the infirmary.[8] In practice this generally meant that the tenants, labourers and servants who lived and worked on the estates and farms of corporation members received tickets and the tenants and other dependants of non-members did not. Thus the infirmary system provided a primitive form of health insurance for those landlords prudent enough to invest in it.

Selecting the surgeon constituted another, and for many the greatest, advantage of corporation membership. Such elections came to be matters of intense personal interest and tests of county politics which frequently brought out many members of the gentry and swelled the subscription lists. A vivid description of the political nature of these contests was provided by Denis Phelan (1785?–1871), a surgeon-apothecary who became a prominent medical charities reformer and was well acquainted with the inside operation of the system. Writing in 1835 he described a typical election:

[6] Ibid.

[7] Denis Phelan, *A statistical inquiry into the present state of the medical charities of Ireland with suggestions for a medical poor law by which they may be rendered much more extensively efficient*, Dublin 1835, 114–15.

[8] Ibid.

The surgeoncy of a county infirmary becomes vacant, or is likely to be so shortly. A canvas takes place by perhaps a dozen or so medical men. The governors, in general are few; and it usually happens, that the surgeon who has most family connexions, or is recommended or introduced by some influential person to one or more of the governors, who have such connexions, is elected. Formerly the Castle [Dublin Castle, seat of the Irish government] and the Protestant hierarchy and clergy, almost nominated these officers. Latterly, however, the local governors take a place in the elections. As a general rule, when elected, such medical gentlemen, from a variety of circumstances become the professional attendants of such of the governors as reside within a radius of eight or ten miles of the Infirmary, which a majority of them do in many counties. The Infirmary surgeon, therefore, is a person in whose professional, as well as private, interests, these governors feel much concerned.[9]

The political aspects of infirmary elections came to be regarded as an abuse in the nineteenth century. In counties not dominated by a small number of powerful men elections were often wide open, aggressive affairs. Various factions marshalled votes for their candidates right up to the very hour of the election. For a time the act of subscribing to the infirmary brought with it the right of immediate exercice of the voting privilege. The packing of infirmary corporations for the purpose of electing the surgeon became so scandalous that a law prohibiting members from voting for a year from the date of their subscriptions was passed in 1833. While doubtless improving the election process this measure had the unfortunate side effect of cutting back subscriptions as well. Subsequently, the infirmary corporations came to be dominated once again by a handful of traditional patrons.[10]

The key to the success of the Infirmaries Act was that while it was permissive it provided incentives which the local gentry found irresistible. Among the most appealing were two kinds of annual subsidies from the government – grand jury presentments and grants from the Irish (later the imperial) treasury. The latter was £100 annually for each infirmary. Except for the period during and immediately after the Napoleonic wars, when because of inflation it was doubled, the sum remained the same through 1851. The infirmary surgeon usually received this money as his salary, although legally it could be used for whatever purpose the infirmary governors saw fit.[11]

The grand jury presentment was more significant. Eighteenth-century Irish grand juries had important and far reaching powers. From about 1750 they gradually acquired administrative and tax authority which transformed them into the main organs of county government.[12] The basis for their growth was

---

9 Ibid. 54.

10 Ibid. 71

11 Medicus, *Observations*, 21–2.

12 For a general discussion of the grand juries see Gearoid O' Tuathaigh, *Ireland before the famine 1798–1848*, Dublin 1972, 83–4; F. S. L. Lyons, *Ireland since the famine*, rev. edn,

the power to levy a county rate known in Ireland as the cess, a property tax which fell on the occupiers of land. By 1830 the grand juries were responsible for the funding and administration of county roads, bridges, gaols, court-houses, piers, houses of industry and the medical charities. They audited the accounts of all past expenditures and had many of the powers of justices of the peace in England. Their tax collectors were armed with summary power of distress and sale.[13]

Presentments were allocations of county revenue derived from the cess. Insofar as the infirmaries were concerned they were more important than the treasury grants because they were increased more easily. Originally the infir-mary presentment in each county was limited to £100 annually, but sub-sequent legislation periodically raised the maximum that could be granted until by 1836 it could, if the grand jurors were inclined to be generous, amount to £1,496 per year.[14] The advantage of this arrangement for the county gentry was considerable. Since the cess was levied upon the occupiers, that is generally upon the tenant farmers who leased land from the landlords, the cost of funding the infirmaries was very widely distributed. At the same time the leading families in the county profited by the proximity of a first-class surgeon and by the patronage involved in their positions as members of the corporation. Their families and dependants were provided with profes-sional medical care very largely at county expense.

In spite of these obvious advantages it took many years for the infirmaries to become adequate medical centres even by what to us appear to be the appallingly low standards of the time. John Howard (1726–90), the English prison and hospital reformer, travelled through Ireland in 1787–8 and re-corded the following impressions:

> The county infirmary at Wicklow is a house rented by the county. It is out of repair – ceiling of the kitchen fallen in. There were nine beds – the bedding very old, and linen only on one bed. Diet, a six-penny loaf every four days, and three pints of milk every day. The infirmary at Maryborough for Queen's County is an old house in which are four rooms for patients – in a room called the tower, two patients, and a little dirty hay on the floor on which they said the nurse lay. This room was very dirty, the ceiling covered with cobwebs and in several places open to the sky. Here I saw one naked pale object, who was under the necessity of tearing his shirt for bandages for his fractured thigh. The surgery was a closet about ten feet by six; the furniture consisted of ten vials, some of them without corks, of a little salve stuck on a board, some tow and pieces of torn paper scattered on the floor. The County Infirmary at Tralee is a ruinous house – the roof falling in. There were eight old bedsteads in four

Glasgow 1973, 77; P. J. Meghan, 'The development of Irish local government', Adminis-tration viii (1960), 335–7.
13 Select committee (1830), 41.
14 Phelan, Statistical inquiry, 20–1.

very dirty rooms – never whitewashed. The patients lay on a little hay or straw and found their own bedding.

Cavan County Hospital. All the rooms very dirty, an upper room full of fowls, a dunghill in the small front court.[15]

Howard provides other equally appalling descriptions of the state of the infirmaries at the end of the eighteenth century. But not every Irish infirmary was so wretchedly inadequate. For example in the infirmary at Cashel:

there are four good wards. The Governors duly attend and great care seems to be taken of the patients. Limerick County Infirmary – thoroughly repaired, white-washed and furnished with new bedding – a cleanly and notable matron. Dundalk Hospital for the County of Louth. The rooms towards the street. The bread good. Proper bedding and sheets. A book is kept for noting down the provisions as they come in.[16]

The obvious inadequacy of facilities and supplies described by Howard very likely contributed to the tendency for the grand juries progressively to increase the annual presentments. The maximum was raised to £600 in 1805 and £1,494 in 1836. Moreover, in 1807 the system was expanded to include some of the Irish cities and towns which were served by grand juries as well.[17] Cork, Dublin, Limerick, Drogheda and Waterford came to establish infirmaries under this provision, producing the apparent anomaly that Ireland came to have more 'county infirmaries' (41) than counties (32). Waterford did not have one but Wicklow had two. Dublin had four in addition to the one at Meath, which had always been considered its county infirmary. Cork had two and Limerick, Drogheda and Waterford city one each based on the county of city arrangements.[18]

By the 1840s increased funding coupled with the construction of permanent buildings in place of the improvised shacks which had been pressed into service initially, had created an infirmary system marked by clean, solidly built and well-ventilated facilities which were well-supplied with good medicines and served by medical men generally considered to be among the best the Irish profession could offer. For example, the County Kerry infirmary at Tralee, which Howard had found so disgraceful in 1787, was described in 1835 as a stone building of two storeys, well sheltered from the winds, well-supplied with water, with ample room in nine well-ventilated wards

---

[15] Quoted in John Fleetwood, *A history of medicine in Ireland*, Dublin 1951, 128.

[16] Ibid. 128–9.

[17] These were known as 'counties of cities' and 'counties of towns'. Nowhere is this arrangement defined very precisely but it is clear that nine towns – Carrickfergus, Drogheda, Galway, Cork, Dublin, Kilkenny, Limerick, Londonderry and Waterford – possessed grand juries of their own. Not all of them created infirmaries under the new law (47 Geo. III, sess. 2, c. 50): *Select committee* (1830), 24. For a list of the counties of cities and counties of towns see the *Abstract of grand jury presentments* (HC 1840, xlvii), 212.

[18] *Poor Law Commission report* (1841), appendix A, 25–6.

containing twenty-three beds. Tralee was, moreover, not considered a particularly outstanding infirmary by the standards of the 1830s; others were both larger and better equipped.[19] But it was far superior to the primitive facilities Howard had seen half-a-century earlier.

Various investigations conducted between 1833 and 1841 collected a great deal of statistical data on all the Irish medical charities, thus providing a firm foundation from which to generalise about their number, size, cost and patient load. Looking at the infirmaries, we know that in 1840, for example, they collectively treated more than 18,000 patients at a cost slightly greater than £40,000.[20] As we would expect, the large urban infirmaries accounted for most of the patients and expenditure. Specifically, the five infirmaries serving Dublin had a combined income of £7,110 while the two at Cork cost £2,619, for an average income per infirmary of nearly £1,400. On the other hand, the average income of the other thirty-four infirmaries was £919. Drogheda was the smallest receiving only £429 while the largest income for a county infirmary was Limerick's at £1,909. The same range holds for numbers of patients. The Dublin infirmaries treated 2,774 and those at Cork 2,099 for an average patient load of 696. The rural infirmaries, on the other hand, averaged only 408 patients. County Down was the smallest with 80. Though basically identical in legal and administrative structure, the infirmaries differed considerably in size and income.[21]

The growth of the infirmary system in the late eighteenth and early nineteenth centuries spurred a number of useful changes. First of all the infirmaries facilitated the spread of professional medical men throughout the country and contributed a significant impulse to the substitution of scientific medicine for the folk cures customarily employed by the Irish peasants, especially in the historically poor southern and western counties. Secondly, the infirmaries encouraged the professionalisation of surgery in Ireland. From their origins in 1765 infirmaries were required to have the credentials of their medical officers approved by the surgical staffs of the Steevens's and Mercer's hospitals in Dublin.[22] In 1784 the Royal College of Surgeons was established in Dublin and in 1796 infirmary positions were formally limited to men holding its licence. Coupled with the demand for surgeons created by the war with France, the monopoly over infirmary positions created unprecedented opportunities for Irish surgeons and led many able young men into the field.[23] As a result the Irish College of Surgeons expanded its curriculum, tightened up its requirements, and rapidly became one of the most respected centres for surgical training in the British Isles. Finally, the success of the infirmaries,

---

[19] *Whately report* (1835), appendix B, pt II, 441.
[20] *Poor Law Commission report* (1841), appendix A, 25–6.
[21] Ibid.
[22] Fleetwood, *History of medicine*, 87.
[23] J. D. H. Widdess, *The Royal College of Surgeons in Ireland and its medical school, 1784–1966*, 2nd edn, Edinburgh–London 1967, 79.

coupled with the recognition that they were capable of treating only a fraction of the sick poor in their respective counties, inspired the creation of a second tier of medical charities – dispensaries – organised along similar lines.

A few dispensaries had been founded in the late eighteenth century by members of the gentry as purely private charities. But by an act of 1805 (45 Geo. III, c. 3) the grand juries and the governors of country infirmaries were jointly empowered to establish dispensaries in places too distant from the infirmaries to allow the poor of those districts the advantages of convenient medical aid.[24] Conceived originally as small outlying auxiliaries intended to provide the deserving poor with free medicines and treatment for comparatively simple ailments, the new dispensaries were not as lavishly funded as their parent infirmaries. Instead of a fixed grant from the grand juries dispensary presentments were tied to local contributions. The act permitted the grand juries to vote presentments equal to the total donations and subscriptions each dispensary could acquire. Thus public subsidy of the dispensaries could never exceed private donations and was determined by them. Moreover, they received no treasury grant at all. Dispensary funding was entirely local. As with the infirmaries, life donors and subscribers of a guinea or more made up the managing committee which was responsible for selecting the medical officer, monitoring expenditures, establishing rules and regulations, defining the geographical extent of the dispensary district, and distributing tickets to worthy recipients of the dispensary services.

The statute was vaguely worded and failed to define precisely what a dispensary was supposed to be. It merely stipulated that dispensaries should provide 'medicine and medical or surgical aid and advice for the poor of such town or place and its neighbourhood, in such manner as they [the managing committee] . . . shall deem most advisable'.[25] Important matters such as the qualifications of the medical officers, the relationship of the dispensary district with others near by, the precise nature of 'medicines and medical or surgical aid', were left to the judgement of laymen.

The Dispensary Act was amended in 1818 in order to separate the dispensary corporations from those of the infirmaries. Under the original statute dispensary committees had been required to request presentments through the infirmary corporations of which they were legally only an extension. This had proved to be a clumsy arrangement. Even in the beginning dispensary committees were composed of local people, sensitive to the needs of their communities, who owed nothing to the infirmaries and received nothing from them. They were in fact, if not in law, independent bodies and as such quickly grew to resent the requirement that they obtain the approval of the infirmary corporation for their funding. Thus from 1818 dispensaries assumed a separate legal status. Their financial position was further improved by a

---

[24] *Royal Commission report*, appendix ii, 291.
[25] Ibid.

statute of 1836 requiring rather than merely permitting grand juries to provide them with sums equal to their subscriptions.[26]

Freed from the control of the infirmaries and guaranteed matching funds from the county, the dispensaries proliferated rapidly in the 1830s. A select committee of the House of Commons estimated that there were slightly fewer than 400 of them in 1830. But five years later Phelan calculated their numbers as closer to 500 and by 1841 a Poor Law Commission report gave a total of 615.[27] By 1839 subscriptions and presentments together exceeded £68,000. In the 1830s various estimates placed the number of patients treated in dispensaries somewhere between 1.0 and 1.3 million. Such large figures are suspect, however, since there was no uniform system of registration. Many dispensaries counted prescriptions or visits rather than individuals treated thus inflating the figures.[28] None the less, the expansion of the dispensary system in the two decades before the great famine was impressive.

Its rapid growth clearly represented the prudence and charitable impulses of the Irish middle and upper classes. But they were responding to important incentives built into the system as well. Having half the cost of a dispensary borne by the county rates was an obvious inducement to subscribers. But there was another as well. Many subscribers made their contributions conditional upon the willingness of the dispensary medical officer to provide free medical care for them and their families.[29] A variation of this practice was that of offering subscriptions of 5s. or 10s. annually, the usual minimum being a guinea, in return for the same free medical care. Both of these practices were illegal since the dispensaries were intended for the treatment of the poor only. But evidence of this sort of bending of the rules abounds. Medical officers were frequently in no position to argue, being grateful for having received the appointment at all.

The distribution of dispensary tickets, too, was a much coveted privilege which lent itself to abuse. Phelan cites the case of a woman who obtained treatment for herself and her daughter though she paid £200 a year in rent on her farm.[30] She had been given the ticket by her landlord who was a subscriber. Shopkeepers in general were accused of subscribing to dispensaries in order to be able to distribute tickets to their customers and thus encourage trade.[31] In some districts well-to-do farmers and the squires were said to receive a greater proportion of the medical officer's time than the poor. Dispensary medical officers complained endlessly of such manipulation of the system by the middle and upper classes but with little effect until 1851 when

---

[26] *Statutes at large*, lxxvi (1836), 712.
[27] *Poor Law Commission report* (1841), 2.
[28] Ibid.
[29] Ibid. 4.
[30] Phelan, *Statistical inquiry*, 156.
[31] *Poor Law Commission report* (1841), 86.

the Medical Charities Act placed the dispensary system under the supervision of the Irish Poor Law Commission.

The dispensaries varied greatly in size and quality. Some were lavishly funded, efficient, large-scale, urban facilities, staffed by the cream of the Irish medical profession, while others were pathetic little country hovels tended by apothecaries or even by medical officers with no proper credentials at all. Many appear to have been simple but adequate buildings containing rooms for the medical officer, storage facilities for the medicines, and a waiting room for patients.[32] But according to one well-informed observer the 'great majority' consisted only of mud cabins or small rooms in very poor houses which, given their damp nature and earthen floors, usually caused the medicines to spoil.[33]

While most of the Irish poor lacked access to facilities as well-supplied and staffed as the well-run urban dispensaries, there seems to be no doubt that by the 1840s the dispensary system as a whole was providing a degree of professional medical care unprecedented in the Irish experience. Within a generation dispensaries had spread over the length and breadth of the country penetrating even the remote villages and valleys of the impoverished and over-populated west and south. While the treatments and medicines such facilities dispensed must have been inadequate by present day standards they must frequently have been an improvement on folk remedies. More importantly perhaps, they introduced into backward and primitive regions medical men who challenged traditional ideas, attitudes, techniques and procedures. The meagreness of the evidence makes it impossible to gauge the dimensions of their impact, but some measure of their importance can be gained from the recognition that once established the dispensaries became indispensable and remained the basic form of public medical relief for the poor until well into the twentieth century.

The third type of medical facility to come within the compass of the medical charity system was the fever hospital. Over-population and poverty combined to render Ireland particularly susceptible to fever epidemics in the early nineteenth century. Severe outbreaks occurred in each decade from the turn of the century through to the late 1840s. Over 112,000 people died of some form of fever in the period 1831–41 and the great famine claimed another half million.[34] In each case the epidemics were associated with crop failures. Fever was endemic in Ireland and flourished when malnutrition reduced the resistance of the population to its effects. Having once obtained

---

[32] Phelan, *Statistical inquiry*, 159.

[33] *Poor Law Commission report* (1841), 85.

[34] Charles Creighton, A *history of epidemics in Britain*, II: *From the extinction of the plague to the present time*, 2nd edn, New York 1965, 278. Creighton's life's work, originally published in 1891, remains useful for its statistics in spite of his conviction that micro-organisms had nothing to do with disease.

a foothold in a region it proved hard to contain. Local outbreaks were spread from county to county by vagrants who wandered about in search of food and work. Periodically most of the country could be afflicted.

'Fever' was a generic term used to describe several different diseases which the medical science of the time found more or less indistinguishable. Typhus, in various forms, and relapsing fever were most common. Both were spread by lice which proliferated very quickly on the dirty and often apathetic peasants who had neither the means nor felt the need to practice modern personal hygiene.[35] Dysentery was frequently present and took its toll as well.

A curious feature of Irish fever epidemics was their reputed tendency to strike the middle and upper classes harder than the lower. Robert Graves (1797–1853), an eminent Irish physician, reported that in the epidemic of 1816–19 'the rate of mortality was much higher among the rich than among the poor. This was a startling fact, and a thousand different explanations of it were given at the time.'[36] In 1840 a doctor in Galway stated that fever in his district had killed one in six among the rich but only one in fifteen among the poor. In the great famine the contrast was even more acute. A medical report from Innishannon maintained mortality among the 'higher and middle classes' bore a ratio of 16:1 as compared with the poor. Another district reported 60–70 per cent mortality for the 'better classes' and 20–25 per cent among the poor.[37]

It is difficult to find a satisfactory explanation for this perceived difference. One scholar has suggested that the comparatively sanitary living conditions of the upper classes insulated them from constant exposure to the diseases and reduced their tendency to build up the resistances and immunities which may have worked to help protect the poor.[38] Whatever the explanation, the perception must have contributed to upper class anxiety about fever and, therefore, may have increased their willingness to contribute money for construction of facilities where fever victims could be isolated and thus the potential for spreading the disease reduced.

The first hospital in Ireland reportedly built specifically for the treatment of fever was opened in Waterford in 1799 on the occasion of a major epidemic.[39] Two others were founded in Dublin soon afterwards but private resources proved to be too slender a thread upon which to hang many such institutions and, consequently, the grand juries were called upon yet again. In 1807 the first Fever Hospital Act (47 Geo. III, c. 44) provided that the grand juries could present up to £100 at each assize for the support of one fever

---

35 Sir William P. MacArthur, 'Medical history of the famine', in R. Dudley Edwards and T. D. Williams (eds), *The great famine: studies in Irish history, 1845–52*, Dublin 1956, 268–9.
36 Creighton, *Epidemics in Britain*, 290.
37 MacArthur, 'Medical history of the famine', 279.
38 Ibid. 280–1.
39 Creighton, *Epidemics in Britain*, 249.

hospital in each county, or county of a city, or county of a town.[40] A subsequent act in 1814 (54 Geo. III, c. 112) increased the amount of the presentment slightly. But the savage epidemic of 1817–18 revealed the limitations of these arrangements and led to substantial expansion of fever hospital facilities and funding.

'Whereas fevers of an infectious nature have for some time past greatly prevailed among the poor in several parts of Ireland, whereby the health of the whole country has been endangered' began the preface to the Fever Hospitals Act of 1818 which went on to create a new category of institutions called district fever hospitals, formed by local subscribers and backed by grand jury grants up to double the total subscriptions and donation.[41] Unlike the county facilities, no limit was put upon the number of district hospitals which could be established. If subscribers could be found, and the grand jury forthcoming, a district fever hospital could be established.

Each such facility was controlled by a corporation similar to those of the county infirmaries. If within the jurisdiction of a county grand jury, its corporation had to include the same major ecclesiastical and political figures who were *ex officio* members of the county infirmary corporations. If within the jurisdiction of a county of a city or county of a town grand jury, its membership was adjusted accordingly. In either event persons with influence and wealth were associated with these institutions.

In order to get the hospitals functioning the corporations were given authority to purchase land up to £500 yearly in value and to build or rent houses 'as plain, as durable, and at as moderate expense as may be'.[42] The sense of urgency which clearly motivated the statute and which resonates through its language surfaces with the provision that once their presentments had been certified by a clerk of the crown, any fever hospital corporation could obtain an immediate advance of money from the consolidated fund. Finally, the same act empowered the lord lieutenant, if requested by local citizens, to appoint a board of health in any town or district where fever appeared. The board was authorised to clean and purify streets, lanes, courts and houses 'and all rooms therein, and all yards, gardens or places belonging to such houses . . . that all nuisances prejudicial to health shall be removed therefrom'.[43]

Other efforts at preventive public health measures emerged out of the same crisis. In 1817 a small committee, known as the fever committee, was formed to advise the government on applications for financial aid to severely afflicted regions.[44] The following year a second committee was established in Dublin to co-ordinate service and co-operation among the city's hospitals. In

---

[40] *Lords committee* (1846), 910.
[41] Sir George Nicholls, A history of the Irish poor law, London 1856, repr. 1967, 77.
[42] Ibid.
[43] Ibid. 78.
[44] Robert B. McDowell, The Irish administration, 1801–1914, London 1964, 167.

addition, government inspectors were dispatched to each of the four traditional provinces to ascertain the nature and degree of their distress. Their reports were submitted to a select committee of the House of Commons whose recommendations served as the basis for legislation in 1819 (59 Geo. III, c. 41) permitting parishes to appoint officers of health in charge of public sanitation. The 1819 act was considered to be an improvement over the measure of the previous year because it defined the duties of officers of health more precisely and made them more workable.[45]

Impressive on paper, at least for the time, none of this legislation accomplished much in the immediate situation. As usual it was permissive rather than compulsory, merely providing the legal framework within which local authorities, working with their own money, could expand their sanitation and hospital facilities. A number of new fever hospitals were built but the other new local powers were either thought to be too expensive to implement or, once implemented, allowed to lapse as soon as the crisis passed.[46] None the less, the crisis had provided both experience and legal precedents which later, in similar circumstances, could be turned to more useful account.

The statistics which survive for fever hospitals present interpretive problems which are not encountered with the dispensaries or the county infirmaries. There were more fever hospitals than infirmaries and, as with the dispensaries, they tend to be grouped together by county. In counties with many of them, such as Tipperary and Cork, they are therefore impossible to segregate one from another. Some compilations provide breakdowns for individual hospitals, giving us some idea of the scope of their activities, but such tables do not include all the hospitals in all parts of the country. Moreover, unlike the other medical charities, it is more difficult to determine the adequacy of fever hospital accommodation. The periodic occurrence of the illnesses they were designed to treat meant fever hospitals were largely empty in low fever years and then overwhelmed at the peak of an epidemic. Regional differences in the intensity of epidemics further complicate interpretation. There is no way of knowing, for example, whether the large numbers of people treated in Tipperary, as compared to Donegal, in 1839 reflected a higher incidence of disease in Tipperary or simply vastly greater hospital accommodation. Dispensaries and infirmaries treated all illnesses (except fever) and, consequently, their case loads did not vary much from year to year. Lastly, figures for fever hospital activities tend to be both irregular and regional reflecting the patterns of fever occurrence across the country. Aside from the surveys of the whole medical charity establishment made by the Poor Inquiry Commission, Dr Phelan, and the Poor Law Commission, there were returns made expressly for fever hospitals in 1819, 1832, 1840, 1847 and 1850.

[45] Ibid.
[46] Ibid. 168.

Fever hospitals proliferated under the provisions of the 1818 act, increasing from 70 to 101 between 1833 and 1845.[47] In the same period their total presentments rose from £13,268 to £22,073. Dependent as they were upon local initiative and funds, it was natural that the distribution of fever hospitals was uneven. In 1839 Cork led the counties with fourteen, followed by Tipperary with twelve. At the other extreme, Queen's county had none and Mayo, Donegal, Londonderry, Sligo, Tyrone, Westmeath and Clare had one each.[48] Dublin had two fever hospitals under the provisions of the 1818 act and two more large facilities funded almost entirely by parliamentary grants which in 1839 amounted to nearly £4,000. An examination of the ratios of fever hospitals to population within each province underlines the distributional disparities. Leinster had thirty-five facilities for a population of 1,869,000, which reduces to a ratio of 1:53,000 persons. Munster had thirty-eight hospitals and 2,161,000 people giving a ratio of 1:57,000. Ulster trailed the other two provinces with fourteen hospitals for 2,278,000 people for a ratio of 1:163,000, while Connaught brought up the rear with only four hospitals for a population of 1,345,000, a ratio of 1:336,000. These figures reveal the limitations of the 1818 act. Local initiative and local money did not meet the real need of the population as a whole. Ulster, one of two comparatively prosperous regions of the country, might well not need abundant fever hospital facilities, but desperately poor Connaught certainly did. These inequities, combined with the continued presence of fever, led to the creation of a new category – the poor law fever hospital.

Following the extension of the new poor law to Ireland in 1838, efforts were made by the Irish government and the Poor Law Commission to bring all the medical charities under the administrative control of the commission. This move generated considerable opposition among the medical professions in both England and Ireland (as will be discussed in chapter 2) which proved sufficient to prevent it for the time being. None the less, the sorry state of fever hospital distribution, which left large areas of the country without any facilities at all, provided unanswerable justification for permitting the poor law authority to move into this sphere of medical relief immediately.

In 1843 parliament provided for the establishment of fever hospitals in poor law unions then without them. They were to be funded out of the poor rate and, in practice, were frequently linked to workhouse infirmaries. Once authorised these facilities expanded rapidly. Within three years twenty-two were in operation, fourteen in the process of building, and fourteen more approved but not yet built.[49] Although but a small beginning when compared to the rest of the medical charities, the emergence of poor-law fever hospitals in the mid-1840s was a portent of the major role the Irish Poor Law Commis-

---

[47] *Poor Law Commission report* (1841), 6–7.
[48] Ibid. appendix A, 22–3. The following analysis of fever hospital statistics is based on data available in this report.
[49] *Lords committee* (1846), 910.

sion was to play in Irish medical relief for the rest of the century. Overall, by the 1840s fever hospitals were the fastest growing element of the medical charities, a fact which suggests that the government and informed local leaders, conditioned by experience with both fever and cholera in the 1830s and 1840s, were by now fully alive to the threat contagious diseases posed to all sections of the population.

Thus, by the 1840s, the Irish medical charities, including the county infirmaries, fever hospitals and dispensaries, comprised some 750 institutions treating approximately a million patients annually at a cost of slightly more than £140,000. For the time and the place this was an impressive achievement. Fifty years earlier Howard had seen only a handful of infirmaries, many of them wretchedly equipped and maintained. Since then the medical charities had become, in Dr Phelan's words, 'the Irish poor law'.[50]

What explains the establishment of these institutions on this scale? Certainly the creation of such an elaborate and expensive system reflected much credit on Irish property owners as well as governmental leaders at both the local and national levels. But it cannot be understood entirely or, perhaps, even largely in terms of disinterested public service by the ruling elite in both town and country. The key to the growth of the medical charities was the grand jury presentments which had come to constitute the bulk of the money behind the county infirmaries and the fever hospitals and fully half of the financial support for the dispensaries. The great attraction of the presentments was their derivation from the cess which, in turn, was collected from the occupiers. The gentry, of course, had to pay their share insofar as they occupied some of the land they owned. But the Irish Poor Law Commission calculated in 1841 that fully three-quarters of the cost of the medical charities was borne by the occupiers, that is to say, the rank-and-file of the Irish agricultural community.[51] Absentee owners who chose not to contribute privately and leased all their holdings could escape entirely though they might realise considerable income from their estates.

The medical charities served the interests of the well-to-do in other ways as well. To be governor of a county infirmary or dispensary frequently meant employing the medical officer as a family doctor at little cost to oneself. In the case of fever hospitals self-interest was less directly served. Yet given the evidence of disproportionate mortality among the upper classes where fever was concerned, they may well have felt that whatever they contributed to the isolation and containment of fever cases was money well spent.

The use of the medical charities by the financially self-sufficient patrons who supported and controlled them came to be regarded as a major abuse in the 1830s. The governmental and private investigations of that decade gath-

---

50 Phelan, *Statistical inquiry*, 9.
51 *Poor Law Commission report* (1841), 15.

ered a great deal of testimony verifying the charge. From 1836 to 1851 reformers sought to win support for a reorganisation of the medical charities by stressing the necessity of ridding the system of this kind of self-serving manipulation. The reformers adopted a strong moral tone and the passage of the Medical Charities Act of 1851 was largely a victory for them.

Without defending this use of the medical charities by the rich, clearly a perversion of the function they were meant to perform, it is probable that without it fewer patrons would have been willing to participate. Local initiative was critical for the creation of both dispensaries and district fever hospitals, collectively the bulk of the medical charities. Local funds and leadership had to be established before the grand juries could be persuaded to recognise the institution and provide it with presentments. The only national money involved was the few thousands of pounds allocated to the infirmaries each year. Under these conditions it appears likely that if contributing to the medical charities had not provided real, immediate and important services to the contributors, comparatively few persons would have done so and the institutions would not have grown and prospered. Circumstantial evidence for this view is provided by the fate of the Badging the Poor Act (1772) which, though based upon financial and administrative arrangements similar to those for the county infirmaries, offered no incentives to patrons and was a total failure. Unfortunate as misuse of the medical charities might have been by ideal standards it may well have been the secret of their success.

Since they first came to their attention some years ago contemporary historians of nineteenth-century Ireland have been much impressed by the pre-1851 medical charities. Some recent appraisals have tended to emphasise the precocity of their administrative structure. For example, Gearoid O' Tuathaigh concludes his summary of the pre-famine health system with the observation that 'by the middle of the century, Ireland, unlike her near neighbour, had a reasonably comprehensive and highly centralised system of health services'.[52] Oliver MacDonagh goes even further:

> If one takes policy and structure as the criteria, Ireland had one of the most advanced health services in Europe in the first half of the nineteenth century. It was to a large degree state supported, uniform and centralised. It aimed at providing the poor – that is, the huge bulk of the population – with some security against both minor and major illness and at rationalising and specialising the hospital services.[53]

In his grand survey of post-famine Ireland, F. S. L. Lyons echoed these views. His treatment of medical relief and public health matters is heavily dependent on MacDonagh's interpretation:[54]

[52] O'Tuathaigh, *Ireland before the famine*, 95.
[53] MacDonagh, *Ireland*, 27.
[54] Lyons, *Ireland since the famine*, 76–9.

This tendency to see the early nineteenth century medical charities as 'uniform' and 'centralised' is overdone. As the descriptions of these institutions provided in this chapter have shown such a view is not tenable. Parliamentary and private investigations in the 1830s and 1840s revealed great variation in practice and efficiency among all the medical charities. Within extremely broad limits medical charity corporations and their medical officers were laws unto themselves. The only bodies which could exert some check on them were the grand juries and they were much too busy, met too infrequently, and lacked the technical expertise to judge complaints and the apparatus to supervise and enforce compliance with their orders. To speak of such a system as centralised, specialised, and uniform because it received some state money, was composed of a variety of institutions, and was founded by statute, is misleading.

The real significance of the unreformed medical charities was twofold. Their very existence by the 1830s, in whatever disarray, meant that the foundation existed for a uniform and centralised system, if only some national administrative organisation could be created to control and direct them. This became a central aim of the reformers. Secondly, the major contribution of the pre-1851 medical charities was the comprehensive nature of the relief they provided. In England state medical relief was tied to absolute destitution, especially after 1834 under the new poor law. But in Ireland it had long been traditional that the poor, a huge and vague classification which included many persons modestly employed, were fit objects for medical relief. The practice dated to the early dispensaries in the eighteenth century and proved irrevocable. It provided the basis for a more generous distribution of medical charity than any other region of the United Kingdom. Therefore, it would be more accurate to say of the pre-reformed medical charities that they were numerous and generous for their time but that by the 1830s they were attracting considerable criticism which over the next decade grew and overshadowed their achievements.

2

The Medical Charities Under Fire, 1830–1846

In the 1830s and 1840s the Irish medical charities came under searching and repeated investigation. Three parliamentary select committees, a royal commission and a private study claimed that there were basic deficiencies in their organisation, financial provision and regional distribution. These revelations triggered more than a decade of heated debate over precisely how these institutions should be reformed. The origins of this scrutiny of the medical charities lay in the concern with poor relief in general.

In the eighteenth century English paupers were provided for by the Elizabethan poor law of 1601 which had established a system of relief based upon the parish. Though national in scope the poor law was administered and financed locally. In the course of the seventeenth and eighteenth centuries it had been much amended and modified to reflect changing conditions and attitudes. While it could scarcely be considered generous the old poor law worked reasonably well under pre-industrial conditions and, what is more important, established the principle that the poor had a right to relief.

Ireland had no poor law, not having been included within the scope of the Elizabethan measure. In the late sixteenth century, prior to the Elizabethan conquest, the country may have had something resembling parochial relief, but the turmoil of the seventeenth century with its cycles of conquest, rebellion and reconquest apparently disrupted whatever local practices had developed.[1] By the beginning of the eighteenth century all organised poor relief on a national level seems to have vanished. However, some efforts were made to remedy the situation, at least in the populous areas. In 1703 Dublin erected a workhouse, or as they were commonly called in Ireland, a house of industry, marking the beginning of direct provision for the poor and recognition of the principle of public taxation for the purpose of poor relief.[2] In 1735 a similar facility was established in Cork and by mid-century both these institutions had acquired the added responsibility of caring for foundling children. Both continued to expand their facilities and functions in subsequent decades and were taken over by the Poor Law Commission in 1838.

Attempts to furnish poor relief on a national scale were less successful. An act of 1715 provided for the apprenticing of helpless, orphaned or deserted

---

[1] Nicholls, *Irish poor law*, 30.
[2] Ibid. 35–6.

18

children but its scope was limited by the requirement that all such children be apprenticed to Protestant tradesmen. In 1772 a more ambitious and comprehensive effort to deal with the poor was devised. The Badging the Poor Act sought to mitigate pauperism by legalising begging for those paupers considered to be deserving.[3] Identified by their distinctive badges, the worthy poor would support themselves through the contributions of the prosperous while their unworthy associates, the malingering able-bodied unemployed, would be forced to find some kind of work. The act also encouraged the creation of charitable corporations in both counties and towns. These bodies were to be composed of leading ecclesiastical and political figures in their regions as well as donors of £20 and annual subscribers of £3. Local money raised for charitable purposes by the corporations was to be augmented by grants from the grand juries. The corporations were to administer poor relief by authorising the licences for the worthy poor, constructing houses of industry for the helpless poor, and by overseeing the placement of orphaned or deserted children in nurseries.

If carried forward on the national scale intended, these provisions might have gone some way toward furnishing Ireland with the foundations for an effective system of poor relief. In practice, however, the act was largely inoperative because it was based largely on the anticipation of local initiative and charitable generosity which did not materialise. Workhouses were constructed in only a few sites. Indeed, the act may well have been counterproductive for its existence on the books, no matter how inadequate its implementation, impeded the subsequent efforts of reformers. Opponents used it to argue that sufficient authority for poor relief already existed and only needed to be acted upon. Consequently, no effective national poor law was established in Ireland until the reformed English system was extended to Ireland in 1838. Only the emergence of the medical charities provided some measure of systematic relief for the broad category of the poor. Eventually it took a crisis in England to pave the way for reform in Ireland.[4] When discontent with the expense and irrationality of the old poor law reached boiling point in the early 1830s the resulting debate bridged the Irish Sea. In 1830 a select committee of the Commons had been created to examine the Irish situation but in the swiftly changing conditions of those turbulent years its report was soon seen as inadequate and a royal commission was appointed

---

[3] Ibid. 51–2.
[4] For a discussion of the problems besetting the old poor law and the ensuing reform movement see Michael Rose, *The English poor law 1780–1930*, Newton Abbot 1971, pts II, III, and Ursula R. Q. Henriques, *Before the welfare state: social administration in early industrial Britain*, London 1979, ch. iii. Also valuable are Anthony Brundage, *The making of the new poor law*, London 1978, and *England's 'Prussian minister' Edwin Chadwick and the politics of government growth, 1832–1854*, London 1988; S. E. Finer, *The life and times of Sir Edwin Chadwick*, London 1952; Sidney Webb and Beatrice Webb, *English local government, VIII: English poor law history, II/i: The last hundred years*, London 1929.

to conduct a more comprehensive and searching inquiry and to recommend legislative solutions to the country's obvious problems.[5] Concerned with poor relief in its broadest terms, the medical charities fell well within the scope of these and subsequent investigations and were examined in detail.

The 1830 select committee was chaired by Thomas Spring Rice, later Lord Monteagle, an Irish landlord with much experience of work of this sort and a member of several Whig cabinets in the 1830s.[6] The committee's inquiry was a modest affair by subsequent standards. It sat for five months in the spring of 1830 and interviewed only twenty witnesses from various parts of Ireland. None the less, it reached some surprising conclusions. In spite of the fact that Ireland lacked a formal poor law, the committee contended that in some respects provision for the poor was superior to that afforded the English.[7] It thought this particularly true for the sick poor and professed to be very impressed with the quality and nationwide distribution of the county infirmaries. In spite of these virtues, however, the committee acknowledged certain weaknesses in the arrangement and operation of many of the medical charities. For example, it lamented the difficulty faced by those many residents of larger counties who lived great distances from their infirmary, and recommended the creation of another infirmary to serve their needs. It regretted that Ulster and Connaught had seen fit to create so few fever hospitals and, while it refrained from demanding the mandatory establishment of some minimum of such institutions, it did suggest that legislation might be necessary if the grand juries in those provinces did not remedy the problem voluntarily.[8] Complaints that grand juries often denied dispensaries presentments equal to their subscriptions suggested that legislation might be necessary to remedy this inequity as well. Most important, the committee had been made aware of the total lack of supervision of the entire range of medical charities and sought a solution through the requirement that all medical charities be required to submit semi-annual reports to their grand juries on such matters as income, expenditure, patient load, qualifications of personnel, and so on, and the institution of regular inspection by the grand juries as well.[9]

Overall, the select committee of 1830 saw the problems of the medical charities as relatively minor; what problems there were could be dealt with

---

5 For more on that decision see ch. iv below.
6 Thomas Spring Rice (1790–1866), first Baron Monteagle, was an Irish landlord, a strong Unionist, and a consistent opponent of Daniel O'Connell. Thought to be a promising young statesman in Canning's last years, Spring Rice was something of a disappointment as Melbourne's Chancellor of the Exchequer. He devoted much time to Irish issues such as poor relief and came to be regarded as an expert on them: *DNB* xviii. 835–7.
7 *Select committee* (1830), 32.
8 Ibid. 26–7.
9 Ibid. 32.

within the context of the grand jury system out of which they had evolved. Consequently, the report emphasised the need to expand and strengthen the grand jury system itself. Of fundamental importance was the desirability of reducing the tax burden now borne by the occupiers by redistributing some of it on to the owners. It concluded that, given the enormous increase in the cess in the preceding three decades, the present arrangements constituted an indefensible exploitation of tenants by landlords.[10]

However sensible and moderate, this approach to medical charities reform turned out to be a dead end. Meaningful reform of the grand juries and the expansion of their administrative functions proved to be impossible. Already overworked, composed of local landlords without extensive legal or adminis-trative experience, meeting for only a few days twice a year – in conjunction with the county assizes – the grand juries could not be made to perform the supervisory role the select committee projected for them. When a compre-hensive new grand jury act became law in 1836, nothing essential had been changed. The scope of grand jury operations had not been expanded and, most important, the cess had not been reformed, remaining fixed on the occupiers.[11]

The institutional inertia of the grand jury system had proved itself resis-tant to parliamentary pressure. Yet the victory of local influence and tradi-tion was pyrrhic. From this period the grand juries began a steady decline as significant agencies for government action. Increasingly they were super-seded in county affairs by departments of the national government such as the Board of Works and the Poor Law Commission.[12] And it is worth noting of the latter agency that, while it could never be considered popular, at least its revenue was derived from a poor rate which fell upon landowners and was considered more just than the cess. The grand juries hung on until eliminated by the Local Government Act of 1898.[13]

The select committee of 1830 had revealed some of the limitations and inequities of the medical charity establishment and had proposed reforms. But its investigation, though useful, had not been particularly thorough and its conception of appropriate corrective measures almost immediately came to appear very tame. In the rapidly shifting political climate of the early 1830s far more radical change suddenly seemed possible. The English poor law, long the focus of popular complaint, was under scrutiny by a royal commission. The Whigs under the leadership of Lord Grey, so recently and unexpectedly come to power and perhaps a little heady with the novelty of it,

---

10 Ibid. 41–2.
11 6 & 7 Wm. IV, c. 116, 'An act to consolidate and amend the laws relating to the presentment of public money by grand juries in Ireland', 20 Aug. 1836, *Statutes at large*, lxxvi. 683–4. See also the valuable recent treatment of the grand juries in Virginia Crossman, *Local government in nineteenth-century Ireland*, Belfast 1994, 30–41.
12 Meghen, 'Irish local government', 337.
13 Crossman, *Local government*, 39–40.

were compiling a growing list of reform projects. Under these circumstances the recommendations of Spring Rice's committee were set aside in favour of the creation of a more powerful investigative body to probe more deeply into the state of the Irish poor. In September 1833 a royal commission was established to carry out this task. Known as the Poor Inquiry Commission, it was chaired by the archbishop of Dublin, Richard Whately (1787–1863), a noted liberal on Irish matters.

This body pursued its charge assiduously. Its members roamed Ireland for two years, interviewing persons high and low, collecting data, assessing the state of institutions, services, personnel, etc. Its reports and statistical tabulations began to appear in 1835 and continued to pour forth for two more years. Its overall recommendations respecting the form and extent of Irish poor relief were controversial and in the event were not acted upon by the British government, a matter which need not concern us here but which will be taken up later. Regardless of the fate of the commission's ideas the data it compiled was more extensive than any previous report. The first report alone (1835) contained ten appendices collectively running to several thousand pages. The second of these (appendix B) concerned public medical relief and had been compiled by a team of three medical men who visited many of the medical charities. Their reports and statistics constituted the most thorough, detailed and objective description of the medical charities assembled up to that time.[14]

Even as the Poor Inquiry Commission was compiling its data, another investigator was in the field. Denis Phelan (1785–1871) was an obscure Tipperary apothecary-surgeon who had worked in various medical charities for many years. While serving as medical officer in a dispensary in Clonmel in the 1820s and early 1830s, he had cultivated the friendship of its founder and patron, Lord Lismore. Subsequently he also became acquainted with the Irish Lord Privy Seal, Viscount Duncannon. Apparently he discussed the inadequacies of the medical charities with these two men, for using their recommendations and influence, he attempted to gain appointment to the Poor Inquiry Commission in the fall of 1833.[15] However, in spite of the patronage of peers he failed in the end to acquire the appointment. Undeterred he conducted his own investigation and the resulting book established his reputation as an authority on the medical charities and launched his career as a medical reformer.

In spite of its title, Phelan's *Statistical inquiry*, published in 1835, is actually weaker in statistical analysis than the Poor Inquiry Commission's treatment of the medical charities in appendix B of its report. His data, though impressive by previous standards, lack the precision and thoroughness of the latter. Working with far less resources than the Poor Inquiry team, he was unable to

[14] *Whately report* (1835), appendix B, 1–32.
[15] Phelan, *Statistical inquiry*, i.

visit as many institutions and was forced to rely upon questionnaires sent to the treasurers and medical officers for the rest. Many were not returned and of those that were he considered some untrustworthy.[16] In spite of these shortcomings Phelan managed to assemble an impressive body of data, analyse it effectively, and present cogent arguments for reform. The book was well received by the London medical press.[17]

The real strength of Phelan's study lies in the considerable personal experience with the medical charities which he brought to it, augmented by his close association with other medical officers and medical charity patrons like Lord Lismore. This 'inside view' provides his work with an authenticity lacking in that of the Poor Inquiry Commission. Phelan's grasp of the politics of medical charity appointments, the role religion played in them and in other aspects of medical charity administration and financing, was unmatched by the rival investigation and report. Thus he provided insights into the actual working of the institutions that could be found nowhere else.

Moreover, it was Phelan as well who was largely responsible for the next, and clearly the best, of the investigations of this period. Capitalising on the recognition accorded him following the appearance of his book, Phelan spent two years in London lobbying for the medical charities bills of 1836 and 1837.[18] His personal contacts with English and Irish politicians and his newly won reputation as an expert led to his appointment to the staff of the recently created Irish branch of the Poor Law Commission in October 1838.[19] At first his duties were those of any other assistant commissioner. He was assigned a district and was responsible for creating the boards of guardians, workhouses and other poor law apparatus in it.

But the act which established the new poor law in Ireland contained two clauses which permitted the Poor Law Commission to inspect fever hospitals, infirmaries and hospitals funded in part with government money. In essence this meant the medical charities. But in deference to the fears expressed by the Irish medical profession regarding the Poor Law Commission, the language of the act was not explicit. Phelan had, it appears, been hired originally with this inspection in mind: he was the only assistant commissioner with medical credentials.[20] Having finished the general tasks associated with implementing the poor law in his district, Phelan began pressing Dublin for

16 Ibid.

17 See the *Medical–Chirurgical Review* ns xxiv (1836), 34–7, and the *Lancet*, 1835–6, ii. 146–51.

18 *Select committee* (1843), 29, 58.

19 Speaking before parliament in 1836, both William Smith O'Brien and Lord Morpeth acknowledged the contributions of a 'Dr Freeman' to their understanding of the problems associated with the Irish medical charities. They must have been misunderstood by the *Hansard* reporter for this could only be a garbled reference to Phelan: *Hansard* xxxiii (31 May 1836), 1207, 1209. Phelan subsequently testified regarding his work in London during this period: *Select committee* (1843), 44.

20 Nicholls, *Irish poor law*, 268n.

permission to begin investigating the medical charities. In February 1840 he was authorised to do so within his district and, upon completion of that in August, was instructed to extend his investigation throughout Ireland.[21] Aided by fellow assistant commissioners and other personnel assigned to him by the central authority, Phelan quickly amassed his data and opinions and submitted his final report in April 1841. It formed the basis for Nicholls's report summarising the deficiencies of the medical charities and recommending their absorption by the Poor Law Commission.

The 1841 Poor Law Commission report was the most thorough and detailed examination of the medical charities ever compiled. Unlike appendix B of the 1835 Poor Inquiry Commission, which was a good but partial survey, or his own book, this report covered every union in Ireland. Already an acknowledged expert in the field, Phelan knew what he was looking for and on this occasion had the resources to find it.

The bulk of what can be known about the pre-1851 medical charities is derived from this report and its two predecessors. However, they are augmented in useful ways by two other inquiries of a non-statistical nature. The first resulted from the failure of the medical charities bills of 1842 and 1843 which led to the creation of a select committee of the Commons in 1843 charged with determining the desirability of reforming the medical charities. It sat for two months and interrogated twenty-three witnesses, including Phelan, half-a-dozen of the most distinguished Irish doctors, numerous Irish landlords thought to be acquainted with the problems of poor relief and medical care in their neighborhoods, as well as various representatives of the Poor Law Commission and its staff. Over 300 pages of testimony were collected. Three years later yet another select committee, this time of the Lords, was convened to ask the question again. Naturally many of the same people who had appeared on both sides of the table in 1843 made their appearance again. Much the same ground was covered, perhaps more thoroughly as over 900 pages of testimony was collected, though much of it dealt with nonmedical aspects of poor relief. Although the select committees contributed little that was new statistically, they are invaluable in exploring the views of men whose experience of the medical charities was deep and varied. They therefore complement nicely the earlier works and when used in conjunction with them provide a large and complex quarry of data and opinion from which a fair estimate of the controversy surrounding medical charities reform can be obtained.

From the point of view of the reformers, the basic importance of these investigations was their exposure of fundamental weaknesses in the administrative structure and operation of the medical charities. These deficiencies they grouped into four categories: (1) the rules on qualifications for medical

---

[21] Letters from the Poor Law Commission to Denis Phelan, 6 Feb., 2 Aug. 1840, *Poor Law Commission report* (1841), appendix B, 27–8.

officers were vague or unfair; (2) the financial arrangements, especially for the fever hospitals and dispensaries, were inadequate and uncertain; (3) the distribution and hence accessibility of these institutions was frequently poor, and many persons who were taxed for their maintenance had no opportunity to use them; (4) finally, the absence of any overall set of standards and of the supervisory machinery to enforce them meant that the medical charities were characterised by extreme diversity which was thought to be detrimental to the welfare of their patients.

It is worth noting that these concerns reflect the rapidly changing standards with respect to effective administration so characteristic of the 1830s and 1840s. By the standards of the eighteenth century the medical charities of the 1830s were imperfect but acceptable, perhaps even admirable. But they did not look so to the increasingly utilitarian minds of their critics. Their keen sense of these deficiencies informed the debate over the precise nature of the reforms to be made in the medical charities over the following decades. Understanding that debate requires closer examination of these issues.

The question of proper and appropriate qualifications for medical personnel was a controversial and very emotional issue. In the first half of the nineteenth century medical science was in a state of profound change. It was becoming empirical and scientific in the modern sense, that is it was groping toward modes of diagnosis and concepts of disease which eventually proved to be more correct and effective than historical practice. Yet at the same time it retained much that was traditional.[22] By the same token the medical profession throughout the British Isles was in the midst of change both in terms of education and professional identity. The basic thrust of these changes was in the direction of greater professionalism and competence but the definition of standards and professional qualifications created a great deal of controversy, suspicion and conflict both within the medical profession and between the profession and various lay authorities such as governmental agencies like the Poor Law Commission. By mid-century government was involved not only in efforts to establish some form of supervising body to accredit members of the profession but was hiring thousands of medical officers to staff various kinds of state medical programmes. This period of extreme uncertainty and acrimony did not end until the General Medical Act of 1858 established uniform and respected standards for medical practitioners throughout the British Isles.[23] The problems arising out of the investi-

---

[22] Roy Porter, *Disease, medicine and society in England, 1550–1860*, London 1987, and A. J. Youngson, *The scientific revolution in Victorian medicine*, New York 1979, provide good, brief introductions to this topic.

[23] For a detailed discussion of the evolution of medical education and the emergence of the modern profession see Irvine Loudon, *Medical care and the general practitioner 1750–1850*, Oxford 1986, and Ivan Waddington, *The medical profession in the industrial revolution*, Dublin 1984. Charles Newman, *The evolution of medical education in the nineteenth century*, London 1957, is useful if now somewhat dated. M. Jeanne Peterson, *The*

gations of the Irish medical charities in the 1830s were part of this larger controversy.

In the early nineteenth century there were three traditional divisions within the medical profession – physicians, surgeons and apothecaries. The physicians were the oldest and most prestigious branch tracing their origins back into the Middle Ages. Royal colleges had been established in London in 1518, in Dublin in 1667 and in Edinburgh in 1681. These were licensing rather than teaching institutions and had been created to provide the public with some guarantee that licentiates were minimally competent.

The education and practice of surgeons were very different from that of physicians. The profession had been linked with the barbers from early times and only achieved independence and status in the late eighteenth century, a step symbolised by the establishment of royal colleges in Edinburgh in 1778, Dublin in 1784 and London in 1800. Unlike physicians, who were internists, surgeons were forbidden to practice internal medicine or to prescribe drugs and were trained basically as craftsmen rather than gentlemen. Under these circumstances a surgeon's education concentrated on general anatomy, the study of basic relationships between organs and structures, and was acquired largely through apprenticeship augmented in the late eighteenth century by six months to a year in London, Edinburgh or Dublin or formal study and attendance at hospitals. It was then customary, though not mandatory, to obtain a licence from one of the royal colleges.

The third branch of the profession was that of the apothecaries. Although originally drug merchants, apothecaries had been allowed to visit the sick and prescribe drugs as well as dispense them since the 1704 ruling of the House of Lords, though they were permitted to charge a fee only for the drugs and not for their advice. In the course of the eighteenth century apothecaries multiplied rapidly coming to outnumber physicians by ten to one by mid-century. Increasingly they obtained surgical certification as well, becoming surgeon-apothecaries. By 1800 80 per cent of provincial medical men were of this category and, indeed, were becoming what would later be termed general practitioners.[24] The Apothecaries Act of 1815 recognised their growing role as medical practitioners and, though it failed to give surgeon-apothecaries equivalent status to the licentiates of the royal colleges, marked an important stage in their professional development.

Although over the years licentiates of the Irish colleges of physicians and surgeons had quarrelled over what each perceived as encroachments on their respective areas of specialisation, they were united in their contempt for the apothecaries. They saw them both as a threat to their own practices and as subverters of professional standards. In addition, they felt themselves to be

medical profession in mid-Victorian London, Berkeley–Los Angeles 1978, is excellent for the period of the Medical Act.

[24] Loudon, *Medical care*, 20–5.

superior to the apothecaries socially and were offended by the perceived threat of an inferior order rising above its proper station. These professional rivalries were inevitably linked in Ireland to the question of proper credentials for medical charities posts. Some apothecaries were serving as dispensary medical officers by the 1830s, a situation which deeply disturbed champions of the rights of royal college licentiates. Henry Maunsell, a noted Irish surgeon and member of the teaching staff of the Royal College of Surgery in Dublin, attributed their appointments not to competence but to local influence and private friendships.[25] From the point of view of the Irish surgeons the situation was made more anxious by the whole question of medical charities reform which raised the prospect that the apothecaries might be granted explicit legal rights to such positions. As one anonymous critic put it, in the event of such legislation being brought forward 'the most vigilant resistance must be offered to every repetition of insidious attempts "to legalise" the admission of a subordinate branch to medical rights, privileges and appointments, for which they have ever been unqualified, and which should not be open to any except the highest grade in the profession'.[26] This problem vexed the Irish medical profession throughout the period of medical charities reform and only subsided in the wake of the General Medical Act of 1858.

Another and even more acrimonious aspect of the credentials problem concerned the monopoly of Irish infirmary positions enjoyed by the licentiates of the Dublin College of Surgeons, a right which dated from shortly after the founding of the infirmaries and which, by the 1830s, had been vigorously reasserted many times.[27] It had originally been intended to encourage the training of surgeons in Irish hospitals and schools, since there was a serious shortage of well-trained professionals in the mid-eighteenth century. Gradually the situation improved. In 1784 the Royal College of Surgeons was established in Dublin and the French war, which began in 1793, led to a further demand for surgeons to serve in the military. This period of heightened demand lasted until the end of the war in 1815 at which point an overabundance of medical men became the problem. Surgeons who had been in the military for years returned to private practice and many new men entered the field. The resulting competition lowered incomes for many; it has been estimated that some of the best men saw their incomes drop by as much

---

25 *Select committee* (1843), 93.

26 Medicus, *Observations*, 20.

27 5 & 6 Geo. III, c. 20 (1765) required that candidates for county infirmary positions pass an examination conducted by the surgical staffs of St Stephen's and Mercer's hospitals in Dublin. 36 Geo. III, c. 9 (1796) altered the requirement to read that surgeons to county infirmaries be licentiates or members of the College of Surgeons, Ireland. Physicians attached to county infirmaries were to be licentiates of the Dublin College of Physicians. Many infirmary medical officers combined the certificate of the Irish College of Surgeons with medical training at Edinburgh: Medicus, *Observations*, 1–2, 18–19.

as two-thirds.[28] Infirmary positions, with their guaranteed salaries and opportunities for a practice among the gentry, were very attractive indeed. But many aspiring surgeons, though Irish, had not qualified in the Dublin college which was both academically demanding and very expensive.

The high cost of a Dublin certificate was mainly due to the five-year apprenticeship requirement which could cost a student up to 200 guineas.[29] The Irish College of Surgeons had developed a school which considered itself pre-eminent in the United Kingdom in the early nineteenth century because it alone insisted upon a classical education along with comprehensive course work and rigorous examinations.[30] Neither Edinburgh nor London required so much. In 1800 the latter required only one course in anatomy and another in surgery before conferring eligibility for examinations. In 1813 a year's attendance at surgical practice in hospital was added, walking the wards. No medicine actually need be learned at all. The cost was thirty guineas. Edinburgh was more rigorous requiring a broader range of courses including some on medicine, chemistry and physics as well as the surgical courses and hospital training. The programme could be completed in two years. The examinations in both Edinburgh and London were conducted secretly while that at Dublin was open to the college and was said to be comparatively thorough.[31] Even the *Lancet*, which customarily attacked the Dublin college mercilessly in the 1830s over the monopoly issue, stated, in what must have been a moment of forgetfulness, that it was the best school for surgery in the British Isles.[32] Faced with criticism of its monopoly the Dublin school reacted by asserting the superiority of its standards and its obligation to protect the public from inferior practitioners.

By the 1830s the controversy over this issue had become intense. Denis Phelan estimated that fully three-quarters of the surgeons practising in Ireland had qualified in Edinburgh or London.[33] He argued that many of these men had years of experience and solid reputations, yet were ineligible for infirmary posts which were considered not only desirable but a mark of distinction. He accused the Dublin college of using their monopoly for merely selfish ends.[34] By the time Phelan made these charges the monopoly controversy was already in full swing. Bitter denunciations of the monopolisers by disgruntled Irish surgeons had begun appearing in the *Lancet* in

[28] Widdess, *Royal College of Surgeons in Ireland*, 54.

[29] Ibid. 11.

[30] Ibid. 47.

[31] For contemporary opinion regarding the various licensing arrangements in the British Isles at this time see the *Lancet*, 1837–8, i. 906–7.

[32] Responding to a query as to the quality of the various UK schools the *Lancet* replied 'We consider Edinburgh the better school for medicine and Dublin the better one for surgery': *Lancet*, 1837–8, ii. 352.

[33] Phelan, *Statistical inquiry*, 56.

[34] Ibid. 57.

1829.[35] Between 1824 and 1836 the *Lancet* maintained a correspondent in Dublin who contributed regular pieces under the pen-name 'Erinensis'. Now thought to have been Dr Peter Hennis Green, a graduate of Trinity College and for some years an assistant and demonstrator to Professor James Macartney there, Erinensis produced a series of articles on the Irish medical colleges and hospitals. Consistent with the editorial policy of his employer, Erinensis probed for evidence of nepotism, monopoly, corruption and inefficiency of every kind. His favourite target was the Irish College of Surgeons.[36] Thomas Wakley, the radical founder and editor of the *Lancet*, was fully prepared to side with the critics having been himself engaged in a protracted quarrel with the London College of Surgeons over similar monopolistic practices.[37] Wakley ignored the Dublin college's claim to academic and professional excellence and championed the cause of the unlicensed practitioners. In a series of editorials beginning in December 1827 Wakley argued for the liberalisation of the college's regulations along lines that would open its examinations to candidates other than those apprenticed to the existing members of the college. By thus abandoning the residency requirement, graduates of other schools of surgery in the United Kingdom and students of non-college surgeons would be given an opportunity to qualify in Ireland.[38]

Wakley's campaign contributed to the reform of certain aspects of the college's requirements. Though determined to maintain the rigour of its academic programme and its hold on infirmary positions, the college obtained a new charter in 1828 and in the following year adopted revised requirements. Students were to produce either a certificate showing they had attended certain sets of lectures stipulated by the college and been present at hospital practice, or, if they had not been resident at the College of Surgeons, evidence of six years of study at a hospital or other school of medicine or surgery. Specific academic requirements were made increasingly stringent.[39] More significantly, perhaps, the controversy stimulated consultations among representatives of the three great colleges of surgery, resulting eventually, in 1838, in the adoption of common standards for their licentiates.[40] But Wakley's hostility to the Irish college remained unabated, largely because of the continued agitation over the monopoly of the infirmary posts. Indeed, in subsequent years his attitudes appear to have hardened.[41]

---

35 *Lancet*, 1829–30, i. 406–7.

36 Martin Fallon (ed.), *The sketches of Erinensis: selections of Irish medical satire, 1824–36*, London 1979, 8–10.

37 S. S. Sprigge, *The life and times of Thomas Wakley*, London 1897, 216–17.

38 *Lancet*, 1827–8, i. 465–7, 498–500, 529–32, 562–4.

39 Widdess, *Royal College of Surgeons in Ireland*, 70.

40 Ibid. 119. See also the speech of Henry Maunsell to the Irish College of Surgeons, 10 Nov. 1838, repr. in the *Lancet*, 1838–9, ii. 317.

41 For example, a typical editorial of this period describes the College of Surgeons as 'a palace cemented with blood' which 'is upheld by the sufferings and unmitigated diseases of a nation': ibid. 1836–7, ii. 378; 1837–8, i. 862–3.

The monopoly issue was at its peak in the mid 1830s. Subsequently it subsided, pushed into the background by the larger controversy regarding reform of the whole of the Irish medical charities system. But it had been important. It had lasted for eight years and had probably done more to focus attention on the inadequacies of the Irish medical charities in the early thirties than any other aspect of their operation. In a sense it was the opening salvo in what was to be a twenty-year battle over the reform of these institutions.

Another aspect of the qualifications question for medical officers in all the medical charities had to do with religion. Two Catholics, Phelan and Dominic Corrigan (1802–80) – a famous and outspoken Dublin physician who held important posts in the Irish government from time to time – argued that Catholics were discriminated against by grand jurors and by the managing corporations of medical charities. Leading figures among the Protestant medical establishment denied it. Given the legacy of sectarian discord characteristic of Ireland from the sixteenth century to the present, it would be extraordinary if such examples could not be found. Surprisingly, this issue failed to generate much heat and contemporary sources provide little evidence that complaints such as those by Phelan or Corrigan generated very much support. The lack of visible controversy in the periodical literature suggests that most of the persons concerned with the medical charity debate thought religious discrimination a minor matter.

A major source of discontent, however, centred on the financial arrangements governing the medical charities. Critics had long opposed the existing combination of grand jury presentments and private charity. They voiced three main complaints. First, the cess, from which the presentments were drawn, was considered an unfair tax falling far too heavily upon the occupiers. Second, private charity was felt to be too insecure a foundation upon which to base the finances of institutions of such importance. Finally, the salaries of the medical officers were too low and too precarious.

Criticism of the cess went back to the select committee of 1830 which recommended that it be levied on the landlords instead of the occupiers. Subsequent investigations supported this view but recommended instead that funding should be derived from a poor rate. For a while agreement on a common approach was delayed by efforts to reform the grand juries which held out hope that the cess could be recast. However, the failure of the Grand Juries (Ireland) Act of 1836 to change the basis for the cess tended to convince most critics that a poor rate was the only serious hope for securing the finances of the medical charities, a view which characterised reform efforts through the forties.[42]

Apprehension about the reliability of voluntary and private charity as an essential part of medical charities funding proved to be well founded. Begin-

42 *Select committee* (1830), 42.

ning in the late thirties and continuing in the forties, subscriptions to all the medical charities began to fall. The evidence is largely anecdotal rather than statistical yet the number and range of complaints on this matter in the pages of the *Dublin Medical Press* and before select committees tends to persuade. Where long runs of annual income figures for isolated medical charities exist they provide confirmation.[43] Prior to the famine the common explanation for declining subscriptions was the sense that the medical charities were soon to be put on the poor rate. Maurice Corr, an Irish doctor who worked with Phelan, explained to the select committee in 1843 that many subscribers had told him

> that they would not pay subscriptions for the institutions when the rates were once laid on and that they considered it unfair that they should be called on for a double tax; and also unfair that some individuals should be taxed first by subscriptions, secondly by county rates [the cess] and thirdly by the poor rate, when other individuals in their districts were charged only the poor rates; and they consequently resolved to withhold their subscriptions.[44]

Infirmary subscriptions also dropped sharply, but for other reasons. After 1836 new subscribers were restricted from voting for new medical officers for a year in order to reduce the practice of packing the management committees just prior to selections. Moreover, increased presentments reduced the need for subscriptions anyway.

Final proof of the vulnerability of the medical charities' dependence on subscribers was provided by the collapse of income from this source during the great famine when the country was most in need of large scale medical relief (see table 1).[45] Although there were twenty-six more dispensaries in operation in 1849 than had been true ten years earlier, subscriptions had fallen by nearly £9,000; the number of fever hospitals had declined by a third in a time of rampant typhus and subscriptions were barely 40 per cent of the 1839 figures; the infirmaries had been least affected but even their subscriptions were nearly halved. Nothing underlined the fears of the reformers regarding the weakness of the charitable aspect of the system as devastatingly as the famine.

Another major criticism of the pre-famine medical charities concerned the remuneration of the medical officers. More precisely, as the infirmary surgeons were comparatively well-off, the problem lay with those working in the dispensaries and fever hospitals. An infirmary surgeon earned about £200 in annual salary plus indeterminant but often substantial augmentations from

---

[43] For example, see the reports of the Rathdown Dispensary in the Royal Irish Academy, Haliday collection: *Forty-first report*, 1853, 12–13.

[44] *Select committee* (1843), 11.

[45] For the 1839 figures see the *Poor Law Commission report* (1841), appendix A, 22–6. For the 1849 figures see the *Abstract of returns of . . . the number of dispensaries, fever hospitals, and infirmaries, for which county presentments were made in 1849* (HC 1850, li), 447.

Table 1

Reduction in subscription to medical charities, 1839–49

Year	Dispensaries		Fever Hospitals		Infirmaries	
	Number	Subscriptions	Number	Subscriptions	Number	Subscriptions
1839	620	34,728	91	7,168	41	2,877
1849	646	25,954	59	1,979	41	1,637

private practice among the gentry. For the others, however, the annual salary was often under £100 and was not generally supplemented by significant private income. Phelan, Corr and other medical witnesses before the various select committees argued that £100 ought to be a minimum salary and Corr insisted that in remote, sparsely populated regions like Connaught, £150 should be the minimum.[46]

In fact most medical officers made substantially less than these recommended figures. Salaries generally varied from £50 to £120 per year, though they could be as low as £30 per year.[47] A survey of the statistics collected by the Poor Law Commission in 1841 reveals that in 1839 approximately three times as many dispensary and fever hospital MOs were paid under £90 per year as made that or more.[48] All too often their salaries were whatever was left over in the dispensary account when everything else had been paid.

Furthermore, the reliance of the system upon subscribers tended to turn medical officers into suppliants, required to beg their patrons each year to renew their contributions.[49] In order to ensure maximum presentments they had sometimes to advance some of the subscription money themselves and then trust that they would be reimbursed. This often humiliating dependence facilitated manipulation of the MO by unscrupulous subscribers. Most commonly this took the form of an understanding that the subscriber, his family and servants would receive free medical care in return for the subscription, or that the subscription might be less than the prescribed one guinea.[50] Reformers condemned these practices and called for a fixed uniform minimum salary which would free medical officers from this kind of pressure. As subscriptions fell off in the 1840s, many MOs became so desperate that even working for the Poor Law Commission began to look good provided that it would mean financial security. The support of the dispensary medical officers was one main reason why the Medical Charities Act passed in 1851. However, though freed from solicitation and uncertainty by poor law administration, the question of what constituted an adequate salary remained unanswered.

---

46 *Select committee* (1843), 16.
47 *Lords committee* (1846), 93; *Poor Law Commission report* (1841), appendix B, 34.
48 Ibid. tables 4–10.
49 *Select committee* (1843), 16.
50 *Poor Law Commission report* (1841), 2–3.

Dispensary MOs continued to feel themselves underpaid well into the twentieth century.

The matter of geographical distribution was initially focused on the county infirmaries. Many of these were located in towns far from the centre of their respective counties. No thought had apparently been given to the problems of access when the infirmaries had been founded. Twenty-seven counties had simply placed them in the town where the assizes were traditionally held with the result that some infirmaries were forty to fifty miles away from the people living on the other side of the county.[51]

The problem was more precisely defined by the various investigative teams of the 1830s and 1840s. Phelan, both in his private study (1835) and in the more extensive work he did for the Poor Law Commission (1841), analysed infirmary use in terms of the distance of each patient's residence from the infirmary. Not surprisingly he found that only persons living close to the infirmaries had the use of them. Of the 18,989 patients treated in 1840, 10,547 lived within five miles and another 4,562 lived within ten miles of an infirmary. To put it another way, almost 80 per cent of infirmary patients lived within a ten-mile radius.[52] Yet the population of the entire county was taxed for their maintenance, meaning that in many if not most cases a majority of a county's residents were paying for services they could not expect to use.

The inaccessibility of the infirmaries had troubled local authorities for some time. Indeed, it was this problem that had prompted legislation in 1805 which permitted grand juries to make presentments for dispensaries.[53] Originally the dispensaries were perceived as auxiliary facilities which would provide for those persons situated far from their infirmaries. Useful as they might be, however, dispensaries were no substitute for hospitals. They had no provisions for in-patients and could not handle persons in need of surgery. Consequently, pressure had built up in favour of expanding the infirmary system, but except for the 1807 act allowing infirmaries in counties of cities and counties of towns, such growth proved to be virtually impossible. The problem lay in the fact that the authority to create new infirmaries was vested in the corporations of existing infirmaries. The law stipulated that if a second infirmary was to be established in any county, the presentments and the treasury grants were to be divided rather than doubled.[54] Thus existing infirmary corporations faced the prospect of reducing their income and effectively halving the salaries of their surgeons if they established another infir-

---

[51] Medicus, *Observations*, 14–15.

[52] *Poor Law Commission report* (1841), appendix A, 26.

[53] 45 Geo. III, c. 111 (1805) gave the governors of county infirmaries and the grand juries the authority to create 'Dispensaries in parts of counties too distant from infirmaries to allow the poor of those districts the advantages of immediate medical aid and advice': Medicus, *Observations*, 2.

[54] Phelan, *Statistical inquiry*, 54.

mary in some other part of the county. Obviously, such a provision meant the problem of inaccessibility would not be dealt with.

The other medical charities, the fever hospitals and dispensaries, were also poorly distributed, though for different reasons. In 1839 there were in Ireland ninety-one fever hospitals (of which seventy-nine were of the district variety) and 619 dispensaries.[55] The district fever hospitals and the dispensaries were primarily dependent on local charitable donations which had to precede county grants. These institutions had evolved without any overall plan at all, founded as they were by local groups which, for whatever reason, generous or selfish, decided to form a managing corporation. All that was required of them was the drawing up of a charter, the collection of subscriptions and donations, the election of a managing committee, medical officer and treasurer, and, finally, an appeal to the local grand jury for recognition and matching funds. The corporation itself decided both to whom it would extend its services and defined the geographical limits of the district. A natural consequence of this way of proceeding was that the richest areas of the country, which needed them least, were most lavishly provided with both dispensaries and fever hospitals while many poorer regions had none at all. Another consequence was that while it was possible for such dispensary and fever hospital districts to have well-defined borders which related rationally one to another, it was not probable. Evidence gathered in the investigations of the 1830s and 1840s showed that managing corporations paid little if any attention to one another. Hence, some districts were defined in terms of the distance the furthest subscriber lived from the dispensary; or some arbitrary distance was hit upon as agreeable to those present at the planning sessions.[56] Districts could be so meandering and indeterminant that medical officers of adjacent dispensaries could pass each other going in opposite directions when calling on patients in outlying fringes of their respective territories.[57]

An examination of the distribution of fever hospitals and dispensaries in Ireland by province shows (see table 2),[58] as could be anticipated, that relatively rich Leinster had the most satisfactory coverage, whilst poor Connaught was desperately short of both dispensaries and fever hospitals. Comparing distribution by county reveals even greater disparities. Wealthy Meath and Dublin counties had one dispensary for every 6,545 and 6,286 persons respectively. On the other hand, County Down, in Ulster, had only one dispensary for every 23,468 persons and County Longford one for every

---

[55] The other 12 were county fever hospitals and received a grand jury grant of £500 regardless of subscriptions. The district fever hospitals, on the other hand, like the dispensaries, were required to obtain their subscriptions before any county money was made over to them: *Poor Law Commission report* (1841), appendix A, 22–3.

[56] Ibid. appendix B, 85.

[57] Medicus, *Observations*, 17.

[58] *Poor Law Commission report* (1841), appendix A, 22–3.

Table 2
Distribution of fever hospitals and dispensaries
in Ireland by province, 1839

Province	Number of		Ratio of population to	
	Dispensaries	Fever Hospitals	Dispensaries	Fever Hospitals
Leinster	192	35	9,734:1	53,400:1
Munster	188	38	11,500:1	56,900:1
Ulster	157	14	14,529:1	162,700:1
Connaught	82	4	16,400:1	336,300:1
Ireland	619	91	13,520:1	84,100:1

22,511.[59] The counties of Cork and Tipperary had thirteen and twelve fever hospitals respectively while Queens county had none and eight other counties had only one each.[60] Critics argued that the result of the existing situation, whereby local people had all the initiative, unchecked by legislation or inspection, meant that some areas actually had too many facilities while others had none at all. The report of the 1846 select committee concluded that while the voluntary system was often of great value in enlisting the sympathies of the wealthy, it also frequently worked great hardship on the poor in the many parts of Ireland where either the will or the means was lacking to originate and sustain enough subscriptions to keep dispensaries and fever hospitals in operation.[61]

The fourth and most universally voiced criticism of the medical charities was their lack of uniform standards. The problem of accessibility was really a part of this larger question. The medical charities had evolved piecemeal in response to specific problems and crises, so that by 1830, even within their respective categories, they had become very diverse institutions, a natural result of the vague wording of the original statutes and the local initiative and money which created and sustained them. As the Poor Inquiry Commission Report put it, 'Under such an easy system of legislation and still more lax administration, it is not to be wondered at that abuses arose.'[62] Up to this time there had been no apparent intention to create a truly systematic, rational and nation-wide network of mutually supporting and complementary institutions. Yet it was by some such standard that the medical charities were judged by the investigators of the 1830s and 1840s. Until the select committee of 1830, no one had ventured to look at the medical charities from a national perspective. But once that had been done, even superficially, it was impossible from then on to look at them in any other way. And from

---

[59] Ibid. 3.
[60] Ibid. appendix A, 22–3.
[61] *Lords committee* (1846), 909
[62] *Whately report* (1835), appendix B, 9.

that viewpoint the most obvious and impressive characteristic of the whole establishment was its lack of uniformity with regard to all of the important characteristics: distribution, organisation, standards and performance.

Examples of the lack of system abound. Dispensary districts were found to contain as many as 33,000 persons or as few as 4,000.[63] One county had fifteen dispensary districts in one area serving 232,000 people while another portion of the same county had no dispensaries at all for 120,000 people. Some rural dispensary districts were more than fifteen miles in diameter while others were only eight or ten, and urban districts were frequently much smaller than that. The calibre of individual dispensary and fever hospital facilities varied from well-constructed and well-ventilated structures to mud huts.[64] In the absence of uniform regulations and standards all manner of irregular practices proliferated. Often no records were kept and those that did exist were unreliable. Storage of medicines was frequently found to be dangerously unprofessional. Strong medicines were found in bottles without labels or, worse, with incorrect labels.[65] The pharmacies had wretched fixtures and were frequently without weights, measures and scales. Some medical officers lumped dispensary medicines with their private stocks thus confusing the two to their own advantage. Surgical instruments were rare and so were leeches, which were expensive. The non-residency of medical officers was another serious problem for, given their meagre incomes, it was not uncommon for doctors to have two or more dispensary districts to serve. This meant they were often not available for emergencies and were generally poorly informed about the health of the people in the districts they merely visited.[66] In times of fever epidemics such ignorance could have serious repercussions.

The county infirmaries were subject to a special form of corruption. Both Phalen and the Poor Inquiry Commission medical team were appalled to find that some infirmary surgeons used the best portions of their buildings as private residences. In County Down, for example, the surgeon occupied most of a building recently constructed at a cost of £5,000 and at the Armagh County Infirmary the surgeon and his family took up 5/12 of the building and had exclusive use of the grounds and garden.[67] Similar provisions at the Galway County Infirmary meant that the patients were never allowed outside in any weather as they might interfere with the recreation of the surgeon.[68]

Examples of irregularities and abuses of this kind are legion. Having once been noted they were reiterated over and over again in the various investigative reports of the 1830s and 1840s. There was near unanimity on the

---

63 *Poor Law Commission report* (1841), 6.
64 Ibid. appendix B, 85.
65 *Whately report* (1835), appendix B, 33.
66 *Select committee* (1843), 12.
67 *Whately report* (1835), appendix B, 450, 456.
68 Ibid. 407.

solution: vest strong supervisory authority in a central agency and provide for systematic and regular inspection. Phelan and the Poor Inquiry Commission recommended such measures in 1835, as did the Poor Law Commission in 1841 which went on to propose itself as the central authority.[69] The select committee of 1843 was so divided between supporters and opponents of the Poor Law Commission as the central authority that it could not write a recommendation, though one source insisted that the committee decided 'by the casting vote of the chairman' to support the creation of an independent medical charities board.[70] The select committee of 1846 came out unequivocally in favour of centralisation and inspection, free from the Poor Law Commission.[71]

Although largely preoccupied with criticism of the medical charities some of the investigators proposed wide-ranging and comprehensive plans for reorganisation as well. Those of Phelan and the medical team of the Poor Inquiry Commission were particularly imaginative and interesting.

Phelan's recommendation was the most systematic.[72] He suggested dividing the entire country into hospital districts based upon population density. Each district hospital was to serve approximately 40,000 persons and to be built in a location as central to the district as circumstances would permit. Each was to have between forty and fifty beds and to be divided into contagious and non-contagious wards so as to allow treatment of fever cases as well as the usual surgical and non-contagious patients which made up the standard fare of the county infirmaries. Each hospital was to have a resident house surgeon who would double as an apothecary, as well as between two and four other medical officers, two of whom at least should be 'operating surgeons'. The boundaries of each hospital district were to be defined so that 'no doubt can arise as to the claim of any sick pauper on a particular hospital, and no delay occur in his obtaining the necessary order from the authorities empowered to grant it'.

Phelan further proposed the establishment of district dispensaries to complement the hospitals. These were to serve approximately 10,000 persons each and were to be rationally arranged to serve the needs of all the people within each hospital district. Generally he thought four dispensaries should be administratively connected to each hospital. One would serve the area immediately around the hospital and the others were to be established at such distances and in such places as were thought to be most expedient. The dispensary contiguous to the hospital was to be attended by at least two of the hospital medical officers. With the exception of emergency cases, which were to be admitted at any time, no one was to be admitted to the hospital unless

---

[69] Phelan, *Statistical inquiry*, 262–92; *Whately report* (1835), appendix B, 8; *Poor Law Commission report* (1841), 18–19.

[70] McDowell, *Irish administration*, 186.

[71] *Lords committee* (1846), 913.

[72] The following discussion is drawn from Phelan, *Statistical inquiry*, 166–71.

first examined and certified by a dispensary medical officer of the district within which the patient resided. Thus the dispensaries were to serve not only as outpatient clinics but as screening centres for the hospitals. The beauty of this arrangement was that the dispensaries were to be functionally and administratively linked to each hospital, the whole apparatus forming one grand, harmonious and comprehensive health care system for the whole of Ireland.

Given an Irish population of some seven million in 1835, Phelan calculated that it would take 180 hospitals and 720 dispensaries to establish the proper network. Naturally the cost of such a system would be huge, but Phelan was undeterred. With some alterations he suggested making use of most of the existing medical charity institutions. Eighteen of the county infirmaries, which had no fever hospitals near by, were to be converted into general district hospitals. Ten other county infirmaries needed no additions or repairs. Consequently, he argued rather breathlessly, only 102 new district hospitals need be built at a cost of approximately £260,400. Since 180 dispensaries would be included in the establishment of the district hospitals, Phelan calculated that modifications to 140 existing dispensaries and construction of 400 new ones would make up the required 720. The cost would be about £134,400, bringing the total for the entire system to £394,400. He suggested raising this sum via a medical poor rate levied on land and urban property. Calculating the total annual rental of land and houses in Ireland at some £15,220,000, he believed a 2 per cent tax on this income would yield around £304,000 and, with the parliamentary grants already allocated for some medical charities, it would be sufficient.

The recommendations of the Poor Inquiry Commission were somewhat different. Appendix B envisaged rational distribution of medical charity facilities, but instead of Phelan's two-tiered system of hospitals and dispensaries, it called for district hospitals of varying sizes. The report recognised the prevailing differences in Irish medical charities by lumping county infirmaries and city hospitals into a category it called 'class A' institutions, while dispensaries and fever hospitals were labelled 'class B'.[73] But it went on to say that 'in every case' this latter category should be assimilated with infirmaries so as to 'combine the advantages of small general hospitals with those of the best dispensaries'. Consequently, the medical charities were to be undifferentiated except by size. All were to be capable of functioning simultaneously as infirmaries, fever hospitals and dispensaries.

It is unclear from the report exactly how this was to be carried out. Apparently the A and B classifications would cease to exist once the general dispensary-hospital system was erected. The report only states that the distances between the institutions, the salaries, classes and numbers of medical officers attached to each institution should be proportional to populations in

[73] *Whately report* (1835), appendix B, 12–13.

cities and towns and to a combination of population and area in rural districts. A general dispensary-hospital was recommended for every city or town of 40–50,000 people. Rural areas were to be served by hospitals of at least between fifteen and twenty beds in districts no greater in area than a six-mile radius from the hospital.[74]

The report was vague, however, on several other matters. With regard to staffing it suggested that hospitals in towns of 5–20,000 inhabitants should employ at least two senior surgeons, two junior medical officers and one resident manager, but the composition of the staffs of both smaller and larger hospitals was ignored. On the important question of how the programme was to be financed, the report said only that funds should be 'secure and respectable', a recommendation hard to dispute. A curious formula for the payment of medical officers was devised. Salaries were to depend on the density of population in the various districts. In remote rural areas MOs were to receive between £75 and £150 per year. In towns of 5–20,000, salaries were not to exceed £100. From that point on salaries were to be graduated so that the larger the town the smaller the salary until at a population of 40,000 the MOs were expected to work for nothing.[75] Clearly, this scheme was based on the assumption that in large urban areas medical officers could be expected to develop large private practices. In such cases they would bear the same relation to their hospitals as the voluntary medical officers in England.

On the face of it these proposals were little short of fantastic. Broadly speaking both called for a rationalisation and expansion of the existing medical charities system so as to create a national network of publicly funded and state administered health care facilities to provide free treatment and medicines for poor persons throughout the country. Not until the expansion of the national health programme in the decades following the Second World War did Ireland achieve a system as generous as these plans advocated.[76] But even though never implemented in the manner originally conceived, the district hospital scheme reshaped contemporary thinking on the role of the medical charities and constituted an ideal which was pursued in one form or another for the next thirty years.

Furthermore, the reports of 1835 envisaged a transformed role for the state in the area of medical care for the poor. The emergence of the Poor Law Commission in Ireland and the debate over medical charities legislation in the years immediately following 1835 refined and extended that role even further. By the 1840s a view of state medicine had emerged in Ireland in advance of anything yet put forward across the Irish Sea.

[74] Ibid. 14.
[75] Ibid. 13.
[76] See Lyons, *Ireland since the famine*, 661–5.

3

The Politics of Medical Charities Reform, 1836–1846

Notwithstanding the insistent demand for reform made by each of the inquiries into the state of the Irish medical charities conducted between 1836 and 1846, nothing was done until the passage of the Medical Charities (Ireland) Act in 1851. But the failure to achieve results should not be taken to indicate a want of effort. On the contrary, medical charities bills in one form or another were introduced into the House of Commons in 1836, 1837, 1838, 1842, 1843, 1850 and, finally, 1851. And another would have been brought forward in 1848 if the Treasury had not stopped it. The primary reason for this record of legislative frustration lay in a profound disagreement over who was to control these institutions – the Poor Law Commission or the Irish medical profession. The latter was fearful of being dominated by the poor law authority, whose treatment of the English doctors was already notorious. Yet neither the Irish gentry nor the English government trusted a medical board to administer the medical charities in an efficient, responsible and disinterested manner. Nor, to complicate matters further, could the Irish doctors themselves agree as to the form reorganisation of the medical charities should take.

These mutually exclusive positions were defined as early as 1837 and hardened over the years. Given the extension of the English Poor Law Commission to Ireland in 1838, the English government saw no reason to create yet another commission or board to administer the medical portion of poor relief. Concurrently, the doctors' fear of the poor law authority was in no way lessened by first-hand experience of its policies and procedures. Renewed efforts at legislation in 1842 and 1843 only deepened mutual suspicions and hostility. Seemingly no amount of assurances or diplomacy could chart a passage through the impasse. It took the great famine of 1845–50, which transformed so much else, to break the deadlock and facilitate a compromise solution.

The first medical charities bill, that of 1836, was the work of William Smith O'Brien, a prominent Irish MP, and was based on the proposals made by Denis Phelan in his *Statistical inquiry*.[1] Not surprisingly, given the consid-

---

[1] William Smith O'Brien (1803–64) was a Protestant landlord and MP. For much of his political career he was a moderate nationalist who took great interest in social issues such as the medical charities. However, despairing of the possibility of acquiring justice for

erable cost of Phelan's system, the bill was not taken seriously and made no progress. Equally damaging to its prospects was the fact that it was not supported by the government. Lord Morpeth, the chief secretary for Ireland, explained that he could not commit himself to the measure as he was planning to introduce one of his own.[2] Furthermore, the question of what to do about Irish poor relief was at that moment very uncertain. Parliament was in the process of considering a major reform of the Irish grand juries, while at the same time digesting the report of the Whately Commission preparatory to the introduction of an Irish poor relief bill. The medical charities and their much publicised deficiencies could conceivably be reorganised within the context of either a grand jury act or a comprehensive poor law. But until the scope of these measures was more clearly defined, Morpeth found it difficult to know whether or not a separate medical charities bill would be needed.

By the following year the situation had clarified. A grand jury act had been passed and, while it had modified the medical charities in detail, it had done nothing to alter their basic organisation or deficiencies.[3] The government's confusion respecting Irish poor relief appeared to have been resolved as well. The Whately Commission recommendations, submitted in the spring of 1837, had called for emigration, a massive programme of capital investment designed to boast employment and the creation of the district hospital network. Historians have found much to praise in this programme but for a variety of reasons the Melbourne administration, then in power, could not accept it. For Melbourne himself the commission's proposals were damned from the start by virtue of his low opinion of the chairman, Archbishop Whately. The prime minister considered Whately to be muddle-headed and observed to Russell that 'It was impossible to be with him ten minutes without knowing that not only can he do no business, but no business can be done in his presence.'[4] More fundamentally, as with O'Brien's bill of the year before, the Whately Commission programme promised to be expensive and it

Ireland through parliament, he joined O'Connell's repeal campaign in 1843 and the Young Ireland movement four years later. He was associated with the hopeless rising of 1848, was convicted of treason and transported to Van Dieman's Land. Pardoned in 1856 he returned to Ireland but played no further part in politics: *DNB* xiv. 777–81.

[2] George William Frederick Howard, seventh earl of Carlisle (1802–64) was known by the courtesy title of Lord Morpeth from 1825 until he succeeded to the peerage on the death of his father in 1848. Chief secretary from 1835 to 1841 in Melbourne's second administration, lord lieutenant 1855–8 and again 1859–64, he guided the Public Health Bill of 1848 through the Commons and served on the General Board of Health with Lord Shaftesbury and Edwin Chadwick from 1848 to 1856. Not considered to be a man of outstanding ability Morpeth was none the less associated with a liberal and generally successful policy in Ireland and had advanced ideas regarding the role of the state in matters of public health: *DNB* x. 19–21.

[3] *Select committee* (1843), 29–30.

[4] John Prest, *Lord John Russell*, Columbia, SC 1972, 113.

was politically inexpedient to ask the English people to spend large amounts of money on remedial programmes for the employment of the Irish when their own poor were not to be provided with similar state subsidised opportunities. The nation's attitude toward poor relief was restrictive rather than generous in the 1830s. The new poor law was indicative of the feeling among the ratepayers that paupers were mostly malingerers who needed a dose of discipline, an attitude which found strong support in parliament.

Finally, the rather strained political circumstances of the second Melbourne government played an important role in the decision respecting Irish poor relief. It had taken office in 1835 under less than promising circumstances. A poorly integrated coalition of Whig, Radical and Irish Nationalist elements, it had only a narrow majority in the Commons and faced an overwhelming Tory opposition in the Lords. Moreover, the government's position in the Commons had been eroded further when two of the most able Whigs, Lord Stanley and James Graham, who had resigned from the previous Whig ministry over the issue of appropriating a portion of the revenue of the Church of Ireland for secular uses, crossed the floor in July 1835 and joined the opposition.

In spite of these unpromising conditions Lord John Russell, the leader of the government in the Commons, was committed to a strong reform policy for Ireland. Indeed, the new liberal approach to Irish affairs was reinforced in that same year when Melbourne formed his second administration in part through a deal with Daniel O'Connell's Irish nationalists. Known as the Lichfield House Compact, the arrangement provided that O'Connell co-operate with the Whigs in the Commons in return for a policy broadly favourable to Irish interests. The most important consequence of this policy was the creation of a government in Ireland intent on being fair to Catholics and on reducing religious discrimination and conflict. Composed of Lord Mulgrave as lord lieutenant, Lord Morpeth as chief secretary and Thomas Drummond as under-secretary, it set an entirely new administrative tone and for six years ruled Ireland without coercion acts while establishing an unprecedented reputation for fairness and efficiency.[5]

Given Tory strength in the Lords the Whigs could not expect to pass many pieces of legislation and rested their Irish policy on administrative change. Nevertheless, Russell very much wanted to pass three basic Irish measures: a municipal reform bill, an Irish church bill with an appropriation clause, and some kind of poor law bill.[6] He could expect a tough fight on the first two, but if he fashioned an Irish poor law which, like the English version, was inexpensive and placed the financial burden on the Irish landlords, he could expect a certain amount of bipartisan support. Such a bill would soothe

5 J. C. Beckett, *The making of modern Ireland, 1603–1923*, London 1966, 314–15.
6 Prest, *Lord John Russell*, 110–15.

the Radicals (who had been crying for some 'progressive' measure) and was personally approved by Stanley. It promised to be one of the few successes the government could claim.[7]

Consequently, it is not surprising that the English government shelved the Whately Commission recommendations and instead dispatched a member of the English Poor Law Commission, George Nicholls, to Ireland to see if the English poor law could be adapted to Irish conditions.[8] To no one's surprise Nicholls concluded, after a six-week tour of the island, that it could be. Thereupon Russell wrote the Poor Relief (Ireland) Bill based upon the English model and introduced it in the Commons in the spring of 1837. The Irish medical charities, which had no counterpart in England, were to be provided for in a separate measure introduced shortly after the poor law bill and run through its parliamentary stages concurrently.[9]

The Irish Medical Charities Bill of 1837 was a comprehensive measure which took account of both the 1835 inquiries although it did not embrace all their recommendations. Its basic provisions are easily summarised. The lord lieutenant was to appoint four salaried medical inspectors who were to possess formal medical credentials and were to be based in a 'Medical Charities Office' in Dublin. The inspectors were responsible for all the medical charities including the lunatic asylums, and were to inspect each institution at least twice a year. All medical charities were to make annual returns detailing their expenses, patients treated, quantities and types of medicines used, and semi-annual returns on the state of contagious diseases in their districts. The grand juries were to continue presenting funds for these charities, though at the order of the lord lieutenant rather than the request of the charity itself, until such time as Ireland had a poor law, when the medical charities would be funded from the poor rates. Dispensary and hospital districts were to be rationalised to increase their accessibility, and, finally, the English Poor Law Commission was to exercise a 'general superintendence' over all the medical charities as well as the four inspectors.[10]

This was a serious measure which had every prospect of getting through. It bore the names of Lord Morpeth, the chief secretary and man responsible for guiding the bill through the Commons, as well as Fitzstephen French and William Smith O'Brien, Irish members associated with the interests of the medical profession. Indeed, for the latter group the bill had many attractions. It ensured their national distribution, substantially improved their finances, and provided professional inspection and administration, thereby establishing the principle that, as Phelan put it, 'the power of regulating the public

---

7   Ibid. 114.
8   Nicholls, *Irish poor law*, 156–8.
9   *Select committee* (1843), 29–30.
10 *Bill for the better regulation of hospitals, dispensaries and other medical charities in Ireland* (HC 1837, iii), 373–82.

medical charities of a country shall be entrusted to members of the medical profession, responsible to the public and government'.[11]

The single significant critical note was sounded by the *Lancet*. The editor, Thomas Wakley, had entered parliament in 1835 and as the 'medical member' (as he liked to see himself) was strategically placed to observe medical legislation. Because he both feared and despised the Poor Law Commission and saw the new bill as enhancing its influence, Wakley opposed it.

Both Wakley and the whole of the English medical profession had good grounds for hostility. The policy of the Poor Law Commission with regard to medical care for the poor was largely determined by its well-known secretary, Edwin Chadwick, one of the principal architects of the New Poor Law. Chadwick was stubborn and dogmatic, lacking in both style and tact, and made enemies by the score. Wakley was much the same. They were well-matched adversaries.

Chadwick's policy regarding the medical profession derived from his view that medicine was a 'sham' and that the doctors were only 'pretending to alleviate disease which if they had the will they had not the skill to prevent'.[12] Consequently he minimised their role in poor relief, and absolutely refused to permit a medical commissioner on the commission itself. He argued that

> on the same grounds that the feelings of the Association [the British Medical Association of which Wakley was a leading spokesman] claim the appointment of a Medical Commissioner, they might claim the appointment of a Medical Cabinet Minister. Medical relief is in quantity only a subordinate branch of the relief, which on the same grounds, would require to be superintended by technical or professional aid. The amount of money expended in building new workhouses or repairing old ones is enough to justify the builders in claiming the appointment of a building or architecture Commissioner: or the attorneys may claim to have an attorney and the bakers who furnish bread and the tradesmen who contribute supplies and exclaim against the degradation of competition and the arbitrary terms of the contracts prescribed by the commissioners, may a fortiori ask for the authoritative protection of a baker or trades commissioner in framing regulations.[13]

Thus in his view doctors and bakers provided equivalent services. Based on this attitude, the approach of the new poor law to medical policy was austere and restrictive. The central authority initially insisted on confining the scope of its medical provisions to paupers whereas under previous practice the parish authorities had often permitted the medical officers to treat the sick poor, a much broader category. The qualifications of a medical officer were broadly defined as 'a person licensed to practice as a medical man', the

---

11 *Lancet*, 1836–7, ii. 412.
12 Finer, *Chadwick*, 158.
13 Ibid. 159–60.

guardians being left to determine just what this might mean.[14] What most galled the doctors was the miserly policy adopted by the commission, under Chadwick's pressure (though he denied it), regarding their remuneration. Medical districts were enlarged, thus increasing the ratio of patients to medical officers and reducing the number of the latter necessary to the working of the system, and the tender system, under which the commission publicly advertised for medical officers and accepted the lowest bids or 'tenders', was employed throughout the country. Salaries dropped to what the doctors thought to be absurd levels.

The English medical profession was appalled by every facet of this treatment. Medical men argued that the tender system was a disservice to the poor and financially counter-productive; that it attracted inexperienced and incompetent personnel or, what amounted to the same thing, successful and prosperous doctors who could afford very low tenders but then assigned the poverty cases to their apprentices.[15] Under such a system the poor could count on perfunctory care and the cheapest medicines available. Inadequate care meant fewer cures, continued poverty and increased pressure on the poor rates. Perhaps most important, the doctors were incensed at the obvious contempt for their profession which was manifest in Chadwick's attitude. It was degrading to be equated with common tradesmen. Eventually the Poor Law Commission came to agree with this view and in 1842 made the tender system illegal. But in the spring and summer of 1837 it was very much in force.[16]

The hostility and suspicion with which the medical men viewed the Poor Law Commission conditioned Wakley's reaction to the Medical Charities Bill of 1837. In spite of its many virtues, which he acknowledged, the entire bill was eternally compromised in his eyes by its eighth clause which stipulated that 'The Poor Law Commissioners . . . shall hereafter exercise a general superintendence over all infirmaries, hospitals, dispensaries, asylums, and other medical charities throughout Ireland, and over the said medical inspectors appointed under the provisions of this Act.'[17] In addition, Clause 47 of the Irish poor law bill, making its way through parliament at the same time, provided the poor law authority with the power to 'visit and inspect and inquire into the management of every hospital, asylum, infirmary, dispensary, mendicity or other charitable institution . . . not wholly supported by voluntary contributions' and hence reinforced their ultimate authority in the whole realm of the Irish medical charities.[18]

In an editorial of 3 June 1837 Wakley began his campaign to stop the

---

[14] Ibid. 158.
[15] Ruth G. Hodgkinson, *The origins of the national health service: the medical services of the new poor law, 1834–71*, London 1967, 75.
[16] Ibid. 78.
[17] Reprinted in the *Lancet*, 1837–8, ii. 375.
[18] Ibid. 381.

Medical Charities Bill. He printed it in full and followed with a critical assessment of its consequences. Using the clauses cited above as evidence of the sinister appetite for power of the commission he warned what the effect must be 'if ever such an odious measure shall be enacted into law, to insult and enthrall the whole body of Irish practitioners, and, ultimately, the whole medical fraternity of England and Scotland'.[19] In conclusion he called for public meetings of the profession in London and 'all the great towns of the kingdom' at which the rank and file should make known their feelings to the government.

Wakley's attack triggered an immediate defence of the bill from two representatives of the Irish medical community then in London speaking in support of the measure, Denis Phelan and Dr Nugent. They argued that Wakley was mistaken in his suspicions about the relationship of the Poor Law Commission and the medical charities.[20] Stressing that the medical inspectors were to be appointed and removed by the lord lieutenant, not by the Poor Law Commission, and that the inspectors were fully empowered to sit as a board and to make general regulations for the care of patients and the management of the medical charities, Phelan and Nugent minimised the role of the poor law authority by arguing that Clause 47 'merely' empowered the commission to visit and inspect the institutions to ensure that they were being conducted according to law. They went on to say that some such power ought to be vested in a responsible agency and that the Poor Law Commission was a logical choice given that the medical charities were to be financed out of the poor rates. In conclusion they stressed the significance of the precedent the bill provided by giving administrative control of the nation's medical charities to the medical profession.

Wakley's response to this letter effectively silenced further support for the bill from the medical side. He excused Phelan and Nugent by suggesting that they had probably been deceived by the Poor Law Commission itself, 'for those grasping despots of Somerset-house are trying to contaminate, with their pestilential breath, the offices of every charitable medical institution in the empire'.[21] He challenged Phelan and Nugent's contention that the Poor Law Commission authority was insignificant by printing Clause 47 in full and calling attention to the last phrase which, he decided, they could not have read. It stated quite clearly that the commission would have the power to issue orders for the 'government' of the medical charities and the officers thereof as the 'Commissioners may deem necessary for the prevention of any *conflict* between the *objects* and purposes of this act'. Or, as Wakley preferred to see it, 'Aye, there is to be "no conflict". In other words the system of tyranny, of oppression, of restriction, and of moderate diet and low salaries,

19 Ibid.
20 Ibid. 411–12.
21 Ibid.

[is] to be uniform. The profession and the people are not to have the opportunity of making any unfavorable comparisons.'[22]

Wakley was a formidable opponent of any parliamentary measure of which he disapproved. Not only did he attack such potential legislation through the editorial pages of his journal, which appeared weekly, but as the member for Finsbury he was in a position to observe and attack bills at every stage of their passage through the parliamentary process. He thus had the unequalled advantage of being able to mobilise opinion outside parliament while observing and opposing objectionable bills within it. Thus, even though Morpeth finessed the Medical Charities Bill through its second reading and by mid-June had positioned it to become law, Wakley's efforts had produced an increasingly coherent opposition among the medical community. It was therefore especially unfortunate for the government and reformers that the king, William IV, died on 20 June 1837, an event which terminated the parliamentary session and meant that pending legislation had to be reintroduced in the new parliament.

It is difficult to judge what the result would have been for the Irish medical charities if these bills had gone through parliament and received the royal assent as until that point had seemed so likely. Clearly, Ireland might have had a truly centralised, comprehensive and securely financed system of state medical care decades ahead of England and other western nations. What is so intriguing about the Medical Charities Bill of 1837 is not only that it would have provided for national organisation and secure funding years before the 1851 Medical Charities Act, but that all the medical charities would have been included, not simply the dispensaries. Infirmaries, fever hospitals, dispensaries and the lunatic asylums would all have been under one authority and based on one tax system. The enhancement of state medicine under the Irish Poor Law Commission in the 1850s and 1860s provides tantalising if indirect evidence that the experiment might have worked well.

The 1837 parliamentary session had had one other important consequence. It had brought the Irish medical community up to speed regarding the supposed dangers posed by the Poor Law Commission. Though no friend of the Irish colleges of surgeons and physicians, Wakley had none the less both alerted them to that threat and provided them with a short course on how to conduct medical politics. They proved to be excellent students.

The election of 1837, the result of the death of the sovereign, returned the Whigs to power once again but narrowed still further their already shaky control of the Commons. Ireland remained the main arena of legislative conflict in the 1838 session with Russell's tripartite package of bills to be fought through once again. He admitted to dreading the prospect.[23] The Poor Relief (Ireland) Bill was reintroduced in February. Eventually, in return for a

22 Ibid. 414.
23 Prest, *Lord John Russell*, 120.

surrender to Peel's views on the tithe bill, it became law. As a result a branch of the Poor Law Commission was established in Dublin under the direction of George Nicholls, and workhouses were soon springing up all over the island.

The government did not reintroduce their medical charities bill in 1838. No doubt ministers felt their problems with regard to Irish legislation to be complex enough without adding to them. Their experience with the doctors in the previous session had not been encouraging. In any event, Russell appears to have thought the relevant clauses of the poor law bill sufficient in themselves to remedy the worst abuses of the medical charities.[24] However, a medical charities bill was put forward in 1838 in spite of the government's diffidence. It was a private measure, the work of Fitzstephen French, the member for Roscommon, who had co-authored the 1837 bill, and at first it was warmly supported by Morpeth.[25]

The management of the medical charities was to be vested in an unpaid board of seven commissioners appointed by the lord lieutenant.[26] These men were to be experienced physicians and surgeons. Another five men with similar credentials, also selected by the lord lieutenant, were to constitute a corps of paid medical inspectors. Secondly, the financial arrangements of the medical charities were to be left unchanged until an Irish poor law was enacted at which point they were to be put on the poor rate. Finally, the qualifications for medical officers were elaborate and controversial. Surgeons were to possess the diploma of one of the degree-granting medical institutions in the United Kingdom, together with proof of five years actual professional study at the institution and three additional years of hospital practice. Morever, each candidate had to show that he had been examined by a board of one of the colleges or universities for at least two hours. Candidates for the position of physician to one of the medical charities had to have a diploma, four years of medical education, and two years of hospital attendance.

To a twentieth-century observer these provisions, though stiff, seem fair enough, especially given the lack of standards characteristic of so many of the early nineteenth-century British medical schools. But these requirements were essentially those of the Irish College of Surgeons. In fact the qualifications clauses had been inspired by several members of that body who had consulted French privately in the winter of 1837–8, though the college itself

---

24 'Medical charities (Ireland): abstract of parliamentary proceedings in reference thereto', Dublin, state paper office, chief secretary's office, official papers (CSO/OP), 1846/156, 1. This is an anonymous chirograph document reviewing past attempts at medical charities legislation and recommending yet another investigation with a view to introducing another medical charities bill in the next session (1847). Although found among the chief secretary's papers internal evidence suggests the author was associated with the Poor Law Commission.

25 *Hansard*, xl (1838), 831–2.

26 *Bill for the better regulation of hospitals, dispensaries and other medical charities in Ireland* (HC 1837–8, iv), 611–12.

was not informed of this meeting and was not officially involved.[27] Nevertheless, the shaping of the bill by the Irish surgeons alienated a significant portion of the medical constituency and was one of the reasons it failed.

The bill ran into trouble immediately and even though it was before parliament from February until the end of June and amended on two occasions, it never got out of committee or beyond discussion of its fundamental principles. As in the previous year Wakley led the attack. In a series of editorials in the *Lancet* in the spring of 1838 he vigorously set forth his objections to some of the basic provisions of the bill. He had no quarrel with its professed object, the reorganisation and rationalisation of the medical charities. But when it came to the composition of the central board Wakley launched into the kind of extravagant abuse for which he was justly famous. He had little regard for unpaid boards:

> such officers cannot be trusted; their conduct is too well known from numerous, long, ruinous experiments. The upright man who discharges the duties of a Commission conscientiously, neglects his profession, and sacrifices his private interests. The majority of unpaid Commissioners either neglect the duties of their office, and slumber at their post, denying all responsibility, and throwing the blame that arises on their colleagues, or they are diligent, and remunerate themselves indirectly by jobs, by extortions or by a convenient oversight of abuses. When some Eastern monarchs send governors to remote provinces, they find it convenient to pay no salaries; . . . but the governor is expected to sustain the lustre of his station, and levies treble the amount of a reasonable income on the inhabitants. A barber without sequins, converted into governor of a Turkish province, may give a faint idea of an unpaid, unfed, Irish Commissioner, suddenly set at liberty among the charities of his country. No man is more likely to apply the vulgar proverb, 'Charity begins at home'.[28]

In pursuing the theme of 'ruinous experiments' of this sort, Wakley seized upon the example of the Irish Asylums Board which had been created in 1822 and, he felt, had probably served as the precedent for the 'obnoxious provisions' of the present bill. The Asylums Board consisted of eight unpaid commissioners. Since 1825 they had authorised the construction of ten asylums, seven of which had been completed by 1833. These facilities had cost the Irish taxpayers the extraordinary sum of £175,605, nearly £200 for each lunatic housed in them. 'Has Ireland not found to its cost', Wakley crowed, 'that unpaid Commissioners are irresponsible, extravagant, jobbing, spendthrifts?'[29]

In subsequent editorials Wakley turned to the second unsatisfactory aspect of French's bill – the qualification clauses. Wakley saw in them the work of

---

[27] 'Report presented to the Royal College of Surgeons by Dr. Maunsell on the Medical Charities Bill of 1838', Dublin, Royal Irish Academy, Tracts, Box 477, T. 44, 1.
[28] *Lancet*, 1837–8, i. 833.
[29] Ibid.

his recent enemies, the Irish monopolists. He insisted that he favoured 'searching, practical, public examinations, before a responsible National Faculty'.[30] But further than that he would not go. He objected to the 'meddling . . . dictating . . . prescribing' character of these clauses. Moreover, he felt the hospital requirement would disqualify nine-tenths of the practitioners in Ireland.[31] It was introduced into the bill, he contended, by the Dublin hospital surgeons who intended thereby to disqualify all but their own apprentices. Consequently, he argued, while the bill appeared to remove the old monopoly enjoyed by the Irish college of surgeons and to share the county infirmary positions with graduates of other schools in the British Isles, in fact its qualification clauses not only reinforced the control of the Irish surgeons but even extended it to the dispensaries and fever hospitals as well. He professed to fear that if this bill passed, it would form a precedent which would speedily be applied in both England and Scotland: 'Every English and Scotch, as well as Irish practitioner, who had not paid a three years' fee to a recognised hospital, will be rendered ineligible to office in an infirmary, dispensary or other medical institution in the empire. The monopolists aim at nothing less.'[32]

Wakley again orchestrated the parliamentary opposition resisting every effort to move the bill through its second reading without a thorough debate on its provisions. Since Irish legislation invariably came up late in the evening when attendance was low he was always supported in his demands for postponement.[33] Thus he gained time and gradually marshalled medical and lay opinion against the bill. Petitions began to come in from various groups of medical men and students in Ireland, expressing hostility to the qualifications clauses.[34] These he dutifully published in his journal and presented to the House of Commons. At the half-yearly meeting of the British Medical Association on 19 March, the president of that body expressly condemned the Medical Charities Bill to the vociferous applause of his audience.[35] Even Denis Phelan was reported to have brought forth a petition against the bill signed, it was said, by the whole of the Irish medical profession.[36]

Yet in spite of growing opposition French pressed on, reminding Wakley 'of a mad knight errant of olden times, asserting to the death, the chastity of a harlot'.[37] In late April French had been sufficiently impressed by his critics to

---

[30] Ibid. 861.

[31] Ibid. 862.

[32] Ibid. 906.

[33] Ibid. 910–11. See also *Hansard*, xlii (1838), 432.

[34] *Lancet*, 1837–8, i. 911–15. See the petition of 48 medical men practising in Dublin against certain clauses in the Medical Charities Bill. Note also the petition of 183 medical students in the several schools of medicine and surgery in Dublin against the bill.

[35] Ibid. 942.

[36] Ibid.

[37] *Lancet*, 1837–8, ii. 87.

cause him to resubmit his bill in amended fashion. By this time Wakley was so confident of his strength that he agreed to a second reading, *pro forma*, in order to allow debate on specific clauses in committee.[38] Opinion was generally hostile to the amended bill. William Smith O'Brien, a strong advocate of medical charities reform and French's co-author of the 1836 bill, felt that 'there was scarcely any part of the Bill which he considered was entitled to the sanction of the House'.[39] The final debate came on 27 June and in spite of French's last ditch efforts to impress the House with the corruption and disarray of the medical charities for which, he argued, his bill would provide the cure, no one was persuaded.[40]

Wakley had won. There was no doubt that this was a personal triumph for him. Both in his journal and in the Commons he had led the opposition from beginning to end as, indeed, he had in 1837. His instincts had been sound. He had instantly perceived the vulnerable points in the bill and had convincingly argued and reiterated in the most emotional language possible that it served the interests not of Ireland but of a small, arrogant, and already well-endowed segment of the medical community. At a stroke he had set doctor against surgeon and layman against both. There was just enough truth in his view that the entire Irish and English medical profession had come down against the Irish College of Surgeons. It was probable in any event that the majority of the concerned Irish and English MPs would have been reluctant to fund a national medical care system run entirely by doctors. But the example of a leading medical reformer denouncing the bill can only have strengthened their resolve.

The failure of the Medical Charities bills of 1837 and 1838 provided an interesting and perplexing dilemma for medical reformers in both England and Ireland. The experience of 1837 had demonstrated the fear felt by the medical profession of any extension of the authority of the Poor Law Commission over primarily medical-care institutions. It had also shown that the doctors could be a formidable pressure group. On the other hand the experience of the following year had shown with equal force that the alternative to a poor law medical charities bill, a measure giving control to the profession, was not feasible either. Of course the 1838 bill had been poorly drafted. It had split the profession from the beginning and that in itself had probably been decisive in determining its fate. But even granting unity of purpose on the medical front the passage of another medical charities bill was far from assured. Opposition to the 1838 measure had also reflected apprehension on the part of Irish politicians to handing over the medical charities to the doctors under any conditions. In the course of the recent debates several voices had been raised against withdrawing financial control from the grand

---

[38] *Hansard*, xlii (1838), 720.
[39] Ibid. 719.
[40] Ibid. xliii (1838), 1148–9.

juries. As one member put it, he would not consent to taking the money from the cess payers and giving it to those who did not themselves pay the cess, and he objected to granting the power of taxing the Irish people to obtain advantages for medical people.[41] This kind of lay opposition to a medical board continued right through the 1840s and was strong enough to convince some of the leading medical men that in the long run there was to be no avoiding a poor law takeover. Since the leaders of the medical community had no intention of allowing that to happen, however, in spite of general agreement as to the need for reform, the outlook for the medical charities remained bleak.

Nevertheless, in spite of failure on the legislative front, the debate over the medical charities had had useful and far-reaching consequences in other respects. For one thing the intense concentration on the whole question of reform had generated a growing awareness of common interests among some members of the Irish medical profession. Of course there had been a long tradition of independence, not to say hostility, among the four degree-granting institutions in Ireland – Trinity College, the royal colleges of physi-cans and surgeons, and the Apothecary's Hall. But faced with the spectre of the Poor Law Commission, they all had a pressing common concern, and the first three bodies especially began to put out feelers designed to explore the possibility of generating greater co-operation. Furthermore, the disastrous intra-professional conflict growing out of the 1838 bill had shown more vividly than ever before the need for unity. The first results of this emerging sense of community were the founding of the *Dublin Medical Press* in January 1839 and the establishment of the Irish Medical Association some months later.

The *Dublin Medical Press* was founded by Arthur Jacob and Henry Maun-sell, both members of the faculty of the Irish College of Surgeons.[42] Jacob and Maunsell were men of energy and strong convictions. Both were devoted to

---

41 Ibid. xlii (1838), 721.
42 Arthur Jacob (1790–1874) was one of the most influential and dynamic figures in nineteenth-century Irish medicine. The grandson, son and brother of practising surgeons he was educated at Steeven's Hospital in Dublin, became a licentiate of the Irish College of Surgeons in 1813, and received his MD from Edinburgh in 1814. After further study in both London and Paris he settled in Dublin in 1816 and began specialising in ophthalmol-ogy. In 1826 he was elected professor of anatomy and surgery in the Irish College of Surgeons a post he held for 41 years. He served the college as president in 1837 and again in 1864. Jacob was an active researcher and is best known for his discovery of the function of 'Jacob's membrane', the layer of tissue in the retina which contains the cells known as rods and cones. Jacob was a highly disciplined scholar and teacher who despised humbug and was noted for his dedication to his students and to the interests of his college and profession as he understood them.
Henry Maunsell (1806–79) was born in Dublin, educated in medicine in Glasgow, and took his licence at the Irish College of Surgeons in 1827. His specialty was midwifery and in 1835 he was elected to that chair in the college. Maunsell's interest reached well beyond his area of specialisation and in 1841 the college made him the first professor of

the College of Surgeons and saw in its rigorous curriculum and monopoly of county infirmary positions a lonely bastion of excellence amid the sloth and corruption of much of what passed for medical training in the early nineteenth century. As the medical charities and the college came under attack in the 1830s they became increasingly anxious about the controversy but had no ready means to defend their institution against hostile critics. The only medical journal in Ireland at the time was the prestigious *Dublin Journal of Medical and Chemical Science*. In 1836 Jacob became its editor and immediately tried to use it as a forum through which to reply to the mounting tide of criticism. But the journal had long had a policy of not engaging in what Maunsell liked to call 'medical politics', and notwithstanding Jacob's importance in both the college and profession his violation of that policy immediately cost him the editorship.[43]

It was very likely the energetic role played by the *Lancet* in 1837 and again in 1838 that convinced Jacob and Maunsell of the imperative need for a similar weapon to serve their own interests. The *Dublin Medical Press* was the result. It was, broadly speaking, an exact replica of the English journal. Both were weeklies devoted to a mixture of scientific and medical–political articles with regular and strong editorial comment. Jacob and Wakley had been adversaries ever since the latter had made it his business to attack the Irish College of Surgeons in the controversy over monopolies in the 1820s. It was therefore probably a source of some irony to Wakley that his old enemy should have paid him the ultimate compliment by founding a journal which in style, tone and subject matter was a carbon copy of his own.

In the opening number Jacob defined the purpose of the new journal:

> To diffuse useful knowledge, and to afford others an opportunity of doing so; to rouse the slumbering energies of the Irish practitioner; to preserve the respectability of the professional character; to instill honorable principles, and foster kind feelings in the breast of the student; and to protect the institutions of the country against the attacks of those interested in their destruction.[44]

For twenty-one of the most controversial years in Irish medical history Jacob used his journal in the vigorous defence of the interests of the profession as he saw them. Articulate, abusive, and occasionally as paranoid as Wakley at his best, Jacob was never dull.

If the *Dublin Medical Press* constituted the first step toward promoting

---

public hygiene in the UK. Active in medical politics, Maunsell served as secretary to the council of the College of Surgeons from 1844 to 1858, a role which required that he spend much of his time in London representing the college and the profession before the British government. In 1860 he purchased a Dublin newspaper, the *Dublin Evening Mail*, which he ran until his death: Robert J. Rowlette, *The Medical Press and Circular, 1839–1939: a hundred years in the life of a medical journal*, London 1939, 3–5.

43 Ibid. 4.

44 *Dublin Medical Press* (DMP) i (1839), 1.

greater co-operation among the various elements of the Irish medical profession, the founding of the Irish Medical Association in May 1839 was certainly the second. Maunsell and Jacob were both involved in that project too, but the major figure was that of their colleague in the College of Surgeons, Richard Carmichael.[45] Carmichael was highly respected and well-known in Irish medical circles and was elected the first permanent president of the organisation, a position he held until his death ten years later. The Irish Medical Association was designed to advise and protect medical men in the discharge of their duties, to watch over the interests of the profession, and 'to be the means of communicating between the profession and the Government'.[46]

The inaugural meeting of the new body was held on 29 May 1839 in the great hall of the College of Surgeons. Physicians and surgeons from all over the country were invited and so large a crowd assembled that the proceedings had to be moved to the college theatre. Carmichael delivered the major address; many toasts were drunk; the dinner was unparalleled in its excellence, we are told; and all present were carried away by conviviality.[47] It was an auspicious beginning.

Another consequence of the medical charities debate was the encouragement it provided for those members of the Irish medical community with advanced ideas on the role of the state in providing medical care for the poor. In spite of the fact that the politics of medical charities reform made legislation impossible for the forseeable future, the mere existence of the controversy stretched the thinking of reformers. The recommendations of Denis Phelan and the Whatley Commission were both examples of that process. Subsequent efforts at legislation had kept the matter before the public and professional eye. The conflict between the medical men and the Irish poor law authority in the wake of its establishment in 1838 in a curious way facilitated this process.

A major source of tension between the doctors and the commission centred on questions of payment. For example, the poor law authority offered its workhouse medical officers a salary of £40 annually. The doctors considered this an absurdly inadequate sum given the demands of the position.[48] Even less satisfactory was the poor law policy regarding implementation of the 1840 Vaccination Act. The effort of the government to eliminate smallpox throughout the United Kingdom was one of the first and most interesting manifestations of state medicine in the nineteenth century. The 1840 act made the Poor Law Commission the responsible agency because it alone

---

45 Rowlette, *Medical Press*, 10–11; Fleetwood, *History of medicine*, 181–2.
46 *DMP* iii (1840), 367.
47 Ibid.
48 For a typical expression of this view see ibid. iv (1840), 378–81.

possessed a network of officials and facilities on a national scale.[49] Vaccination had been provided by some Irish doctors in the past, but the 1840 act was designed to systematise the practice and make it free. Under the provisions of the act the Poor Law commission was authorised to hire doctors to perform the service at an annual rate of 1s. per patient through the first 200 cases and 6d. per patient thereafter.[50]

The Irish doctors were appalled at these terms. They considered the sums insultingly small.[51] Their irritation was compounded by the knowledge that English doctors were paid at a higher rate, 1s. 6d. per case.[52] Moreover, the halving of the rate after 200 cases was not only candle-end mentality, so typical of the approach of the Poor Law Commission, but probably counter-productive as well. It discouraged doctors from vaccinating more than 200 persons per year. Critics charged that the opposite approach should have been employed. Vaccinators should have been paid proportionally more the greater the number of persons they immunised. That would have encouraged the vaccination of the entire population, presumably the purpose of the act. But the reasoning behind the 1840 arrangement had nothing to do with public health, rather it reflected the ideas on economy characteristic of the ratepayers and Boards of Guardians. Moreover, the rate of payment for each vaccination, small as it was, was only a maximum set by the Poor Law Commission. The guardians could arrange for less if they could find a doctor to accept such fees – the tender system again. Naturally the Irish medical profession was vocal in its opposition. A series of editorials in the *Dublin Medical Press* denounced the act and the Poor Law Commission in highly emotional language.[53] Throughout provincial Ireland practitioners met to discuss and condemn these developments. Resolutions were passed and petitions were submitted to the government, none of which did any good. The act was implemented without major amendment. It was not a success. Witnesses before the select committees of 1843 and 1846 testified to the effect that not only was the Vaccination Act a disaster, but that its handling embittered the doctors against the Poor Law Commission.[54] Their first encounter had only served to reinforce the worst fears of the Irish medical community. In this climate of opinion rumours flourished. There was much talk about the likely takeover of the entire medical charity establishment under the provisions of the notorious Clause 47 of the Irish poor law act.[55] In addition some critics speculated that the commission sought to acquire

[49] R. J. Lambert, 'A Victorian national health service: state vaccination, 1855–71', *Historical Journal* v (1962), 2.

[50] Nicholls, *Irish poor law*, 268.

[51] Testimony of Henry Maunsell, *Select committee* (1843), 284.

[52] Ibid. See also Hodgkinson, *Origins*, 126.

[53] See particularly *DMP* iv (1840), 347–8, 360–1.

[54] Testimony of M. D. Nugent, W. L. Kidd, Richard Corbett and Henry Maunsell, *Select committee* (1843), 37–8, 98, 189, 284.

[55] *DMP* iii–iv (1840, 1841), passim.

authority to enforce sanitary legislation as well, that it saw itself as a board of health. These developments and rumours fuelled wide-ranging debate on all aspects of the proper role of the state with respect to medical care and public health.

In January 1839 Henry Maunsell addressed these matters in a speech to the College of Surgeons in Dublin. Focusing on the theme 'political medicine', he argued that it involved far more than an aggressive and informed defence of the interests of the profession. He suggested that it involved shifting one's focus from treatment of individuals to the higher goal of protecting public health and providing for the welfare of the community as a whole.[56] Emphasising the need for effective preventive measures he argued that widespread and generous provision of medical care for the poor should be one of the main goals of every well-ordered society. He lamented the fact that the medical profession had taken so little interest in these matters that, as a consequence of their neglect, preventative measures were frequently poorly conceived and executed. Faced with an epidemic, boards of health had to be improvised and were usually staffed by inexperienced personnel who were frequently incompetent and uncertain of how best to proceed. Maunsell contended that too little authority and organisation existed on the national level to deal with these emergencies effectively. Unsanitary conditions were allowed to persist in the cities and towns because no medical board had the powers to deal with them. He concluded with the warning that if the medical profession did not pay greater attention to these questions they would soon find the Poor Law Commission as the public health authority and themselves barred from playing their proper role.

Delivered some three years prior to the appearance of Edwin Chadwick's seminal *Report on the sanitary condition of the labouring population of Great Britain* (1842), Maunsell's analysis illustrates the way the Irish debates over medical charity reform advanced the conception of the role of state medicine. In the following month Denis Phelan spoke on the desirability of putting the medical charities on the firmer ground of the poor rate. This was common fare by this time but what was interesting was his reason. 'We all know', Phelan said, 'that sickness creates poverty' and went on to argue for support of the medical charities as institutions of poverty prevention superior to workhouses because the latter only housed individuals and families already broken by disease and malnutrition.[57]

In an editorial of September 1841, addressed specifically to the inequities of the much despised tender system, Arthur Jacob was moved to argue for something rather like the National Health Service:

> When the state undertakes to preserve the health of life of a subject, the means afforded must be unlimited. We must have no 'farming' of the sick, no

---

[56] Ibid. i (1839), 65–6.
[57] Ibid. 74.

'contracts' for wholesale doctoring, no providing of relief 'on the lowest terms'.
. . . If general relief is to be administered in conformity with preconceived
fixed principles, medical relief must be afforded with a fixed principle also,
and that principle we insist upon it, must be that if the state undertakes the
treatment of a patient with a view to the preservation of his life, everything
that can be done should be done.[58]

By 1841, a year before the public health movement started in England, the
theory that sickness caused poverty and that the state had to do something
substantial about it was clearly formulated in Ireland. In that same year the
Irish College of Surgeons created the first chair of public health in the British
Isles and Henry Maunsell was invited to occupy it. The Irish doctors were far
from victory in their struggle with the Poor Law Commission but they were
well on the way to developing a theory of state medicine in which they
played a far more important role than a sanitarian like Chadwick had yet
imagined, a role, indeed, which smacked more of the twentieth century than
the nineteenth.

In 1842 and 1843 further efforts were made to place the medical charities
on a sounder footing. The first grew out of the renewed attempt of the Poor
Law Commission to reorganise and absorb those institutions. In 1840, its
authority and administrative apparatus now established throughout the island, the commission turned its attention to the medical charities whose
financial condition had not improved in the years since the highly critical
reports of the mid-thirties. As we have seen, responsibility for investigating
and reporting upon their condition fell to Denis Phelan, who had been
appointed to the commission shortly after its extension to Ireland. With the
resources and the authority of the government behind him, Phelan conducted his investigation. He submitted his findings to George Nicholls, head
of the Irish division of the Poor Law Commission in 1841 and the latter
promptly framed a medical charities bill which was placed before parliament
in the spring of the following year.[59]

Nicholls proposed to put the dispensaries and fever hospitals on the poor
rate and to bring their administration directly under the direction of the Poor
Law Commission. Dispensary and fever hospital districts were to be created
in each union composed of appropriate numbers of electoral divisions, the
rating units of the Irish unions. Each institution was to be administered
directly by a managing committee composed of wardens of the electoral
divisions, the guardians resident in each district, local clergy and a number of
locals elected from among the ratepayers. In regions now more than twenty
miles from existing county infirmaries the bill provided for the creation of
district hospitals which were to fulfill the same function as the infirmaries. A
Medical Charities Board composed of between five and seven eminent repre-

---

[58] Ibid. vi (1841), 206.
[59] *Poor Law Commission report* (1841), 14–20.

sentatives of the profession, resident in the Dublin area, was to be created to advise the Poor Law Commission. A number of medical inspectors were to be appointed to oversee the operation of the medical facilities and to maintain liaison between them and the central board.

There were a number of interesting and novel features to this bill. Fore-most among them was the fact that the county infirmaries had been left out. Nicholls argued that the infirmaries were better off financially than the rest of the medical charities and that they were more effectively controlled by the grand juries. He also suggested that the Poor Law Commission already pos-sessed certain powers with respect to the infirmaries which he hoped would be sufficient to remedy existing abuses and secure their good management in the future. Thus he apparently hoped to placate the politically powerful infirmary surgeons before the battle began. Secondly, Phelan's influence is manifest throughout the proposal, most strikingly with the inclusion of the district hospitals which in combination with the other institutions would nearly create his 1835 scheme. Finally, there was to be no ambiguity as to who was to run the reorganised medical charities. Nicholls made it clear from the outset that the proposed medical board's function was purely advisory. Its members were to be paid a nominal sum, two guineas per meeting, the inspectors were to be appointed by the lord lieutenant, and in the event of disagreement between it and the Poor Law Board the ruling of the latter was to be final.

Throughout the spring and early summer medical circles in Ireland buzzed with discussion and rumour. As was to be expected, the *Dublin Medical Press* set a strongly hostile tone from the start. In a series of editorials beginning in April and running through to the end of June, the bill was subjected to searching and scathing criticism along familiar lines.[60] From the perspective of the journal the leading villains in this affair were Nicholls and Phelan. The latter was portrayed as an eminence grise working behind the scenes in an effort to raise the Poor Law Commission and hence himself over the medical profession he had not the credentials to belong to otherwise. Of course Phelan was an apothecary-surgeon. But his surgeon's licence was from London and Jacob and his colleagues at the Irish College of Surgeons never took it seriously. The *DMP* never failed to refer to him as an apothecary or to note the 'smell of rhubarb' about all with which he was engaged.

Indeed Phelan was a more serious antagonist than poor Nicholls. The latter was an easy target: he was English, new to Ireland, and the author of the poor law machinery which was fast becoming so unpopular around the island. Phelan, on the other hand, was native Irish, something of a national-ist, a member of the medical profession with a following among the provin-cial medical officers, and a man with a growing reputation as a medical charities reformer. Snide references to his credentials by the *DMP* could be a

60 *DMP* viii (1842), 238–9, 254–5, 286–7, 300–2.

positive advantage in provincial medical circles where the influence, prestige and prosperity of the Dublin medical elite were profoundly resented.

However, the *DMP* was energetic in its efforts to defeat the measure and found evidence of sloppiness in the way in which Phelan had collected his information. In the now familiar run of aggressive editorials they weakened his credibility by implying, with some plausibility, that he and his Poor Law Commission superiors had cooked the numbers in order to strengthen their case for takeover.[61] The result of the affair was a public dressing down for the Poor Law Commission. Nicholls was charged by members of the House of Lords with having deceived the government.[62] It was hardly an auspicious moment to request the kind of expansion of responsibility and operations involved in taking over the medical charities. The *DMP* was elated.[63]

Meanwhile the Irish medical delegation which had met the Poor Law Commission in London in the spring had been busy contriving a proposal more suitable to the medical profession than that of Nicholls. Entitled 'A draft of suggestions for a medical charities bill', it incorporated exactly the changes one would expect.[64] Instead of vesting control in the Poor Law Commission, the proposed bill placed it in the hands of the lord lieutenant and a central medical board. The medical charities were still to be financed out of the poor rates but the Poor Law Commission was to have only collecting and auditing authority over that portion of the rates allocated to the medical charities.[65] The proposed medical board was to be composed of nine members including the chief secretary, the president and two members of the College of Physicians, the president and two members of the College of Surgeons, and the governor and one member of the Apothecary's Hall. The board would have complete authority to determine the qualifications of all applicants to medical charities positions.

In many ways this bill reflected greater co-operation and planning among the various elements of the Irish medical profession than any of its predecessors. Even the apothecaries were included. Nevertheless, it soon became apparent that the profession was not completely behind the Dublin colleges and the editorial policy of the *DMP*. No sooner had the new proposal been submitted to the government in May than a dissenting note was sounded by two Dublin physicians of considerable stature – Dominic Corrigan and Robert Harrison.[66]

Corrigan and Harrison contested virtually every aspect of the 'Draft of

---

[61] *Hansard*, lxiv (1842), 694–700.
[62] Ibid.
[63] *DMP* viii (1842), 11.
[64] Testimony of Henry Maunsell, *Select committee* (1843), 290.
[65] Robert Harrison and Dominic Corrigan, 'Observations on the draft of a bill for the regulation and support of medical charities in Ireland', Royal Irish Academy, Haliday pamphlet collection, no. 1833, 2–10.
[66] Ibid.

suggestions', but their main concern was the effect of concentrating so much power in the hands of representatives of the Dublin colleges. Corrigan and Harrison made proposals of their own which in general were much closer to those of Nicholls. The crux of their plan was the entire elimination of the board, arguing that it could be dispensed with if the duties of the medical inspectors were properly defined and efficiently performed.[67] Corrigan and Harrison included a massive sample of opinions on their ideas obtained from medical officers all over the island. This array of opinion illustrated the great variety of reactions to the various reform proposals characteristic of the provincial medical establishment and decisively undermined the assertions of the DMP that the entire profession was set against the Poor Law Commission plans for the reorganisation of the medical charities. To a certain extent Corrigan and Harrison restored the perspective on the problems and dangers of reform which had been lost in the general discrediting of Phelan and Nicholls. The two Dublin physicans were able to criticise the Irish medical establishment with a credibility denied agents of the despised Poor Law Commission. They spoke for the many provincial medical men who feared that a central board responsible to no one but the lord lieutenant would inevitably favour its own students and friends to the exclusion of nearly everyone else. The DMP railed against Corrigan and Harrison calling them dupes of the Poor Law Commission, but such charges could not disguise the fact that as in 1838 the profession was profoundly split regarding medical charities reform.

In August Lord Eliot, the Chief Secretary in Sir Robert Peel's government, finally brought in his medical charities bill.[68] Throughout the autumn of 1842 the DMP took Eliot's bill apart clause by clause in a repetition of its editorials of the spring.[69] Both sides marshalled what support they could. Across the country the doctors met, argued and petitioned for or against the bill. Eliot tried to demonstrate that the DMP represented only the elite of the colleges and profession.[70] But Harrison, Corrigan and their supporters not-withstanding, it became increasingly clear in the early winter that the DMP in fact had the best of it. While far from unanimous, provincial support also ran strongly against the bill. The fact that the DMP was the only voice for the profession on the island dealing with such issues gave it a tremendous advantage and Jacob and Maunsell used it effectively. In January Eliot admit-ted defeat. He lacked the votes to get the bill through parliament and withdrew it. In a characteristic move the DMP promptly forgave him his role in the whole affair.[71] The medical establishment did not like to alienate chief

---

67 Ibid.
68 *Bill for the better regulation and support of medical charities in Ireland* (HC 1842, iii), 191–216.
69 DMP viii (1842), 129–38, 171–4, 188–9, 206–7, 219–21, 237–8, 251–3.
70 Ibid. 363.
71 Ibid. ix (1843) 45–6.

secretaries and preferred to see them as victims of their advisors whenever they could. In this case it was easy. They blamed everything on the Poor Law Commission.

With the failure of a government measure Fitzstephens French surfaced once again with another bill of his own which favoured the medical profession and generally had its support.[72] The government opposed it, advised to do so by the Poor Law Commission.[73] Under those circumstances the new bill had no chance and so, in return for a promise to convene a select committee to consider the problems of the medical charities, French withdrew his measure too.

The committee duly met. It was composed of many of the most prominent Irish politicians: French, of course, and Eliot as well as W. S. O'Brien, and two men who would eventually become chief secretaries and play an important role in the development of the medical charities, John Young and William Somerville.[74] The committee sat continuously for two months during which time a mass of evidence was produced from peers, members of parliament and all the leaders of the medical profession in Ireland. Nothing emerged that had not been clear before. However, the tone of the investigation was less emotional than the debates on the failed Medical Charities bills had been. The committee's report underlined the fundamental differences between the Poor Law Commission and the government on the one hand and the Irish doctors on the other. The continued decline in voluntary subscriptions in the years immediately following kept the question of medical charities reform alive. In 1846 another select committee was convened, in part in response to the increasing urgency that was felt on the question. The committee went over the same ground and revealed the same deadlock. It seemed at that time that the stalemate would go on indefinitely. But a breakthrough of sorts was just around the corner. As the committee met in the spring of 1846 the first serious effects of the failure of the potato crop in the previous summer were beginning to be felt. The great famine had begun. It was to change a great many things in Ireland, the medical charities among them.

---

[72] *Bill for the better regulation and support of medical charities in Ireland* (HC 1843, iii), 383–402.
[73] 'Medical charities', CSO/OP, 1846/156, 3–4.
[74] Ibid. 4–5. Sir William Somerville (1802–73) was chief secretary from 1847 to 1852 and as such had to deal with the worst phase of the famine. He was the person most responsible for the passage of the Medical Charities Act in 1851. Sir John Young (1807–76) was chief secretary from 1852 to 1855 and was involved in the last serious attempt by the Irish Poor Law Commission to gain control of the county infirmaries.

4

The Famine and the Passage of the Medical Charities (Ireland) Act, 1851

Of all the countries of western Europe Ireland was the most vulnerable to massive famine in the 1840s. Its population had swollen to over eight million persons, almost twice its present size.[1] Furthermore, it is estimated that fully one-third of those people were absolutely dependent upon potatoes for their existence and that an even larger percentage was at least partially dependent on the same crop.[2] The reliability of the potato crop had never been certain. Significant failures had occurred periodically throughout the eighteenth and early nineteenth centuries causing widespread distress but had not been severe enough to interrupt the constant demographic growth. The great famine was an entirely different matter and due to the magnitude of its impact has come to be seen as a fundamental watershed in Irish history.[3]

The famine began in the summer of 1845 when a new potato disease, first noted in North America and then later on the Continent and in England, made its appearance in Waterford and Wexford. It was a form of blight caused by a fungus which affected both the plant and the potatoes themselves. Its spread and occurrence in Ireland in the late 1840s was uneven but cumulatively devastating. In 1845 the potato crop was very heavy and about a sixth of it had been harvested before the disease struck. Thus, although the blight eventually spread to seventeen counties and produced severe hardship, the entire country was not affected and the failure of the crop was not complete.[4] At first the situation therefore seemed to resemble many that had occurred in the immediate past. But in 1846 the spring and summer were once again unusually wet and the crop was a total loss. This was unprecedented and many of the Irish labourers, already weakened by the previous failure and having consumed much of what stores they had set aside for such eventualities, were in desperate straits. The 1847 crop was not seriously affected by the blight but the yield was small owing to the fact that many people had failed to plant their fields in the spring because of illness, despair, or consumption of their seed potatoes. 1848 brought another total failure of

---

[1] O Grada, 'Poverty, population, and agriculture', 118.
[2] Ibid. 112.
[3] Foster takes a different view, arguing that 1815 was more important as a watershed than 1845: Foster, *Modern Ireland*, 318.
[4] James S. Donnelly, Jr, 'Famine and government response, 1845–46', in Vaughn, *Ireland Under the union*, I: 1801–70, 272–3.

crop, and 1849 and 1850 partial failures, but by then the blight was on the wane and the class of people it could hurt largely gone. It was this sequence of partial and total failures, particularly in the years 1845–8, that produced the catastrophic loss of life and massive emigration forever associated with this disaster.

According to the census of 1841 the Irish population was 8,175,124. By 1851 it was 6,552,386, a decline of approximately 20 per cent.[5] It is not possible to give precise figures on how many died and how many emigrated. Some authorities suggest that due to resistance to registration on the part of the rural Irish the 1841 census was too low. They also argue that natural increase should have produced a figure of approximately nine million persons by 1851. Consequently, the loss in population is thought to stand at around two-and-a-half million. Of these one-and-a-half million emigrated, most of them to North America. The rest, between 800,000 and 1,000,000 persons, died during the famine, many perishing in remote villages and valleys and hence never recorded in the mortality figures.[6]

The burden of suffering was unevenly distributed within Ireland both geographically and socially. The hardest hit areas were the very poor and densely populated counties of the west and south. Between 1841 and 1851 the population of Connaught fell by 29 per cent, that of Munster by 22 per cent, of Ulster by 16 per cent, and of Leinster by 15 per cent.[7] The lowest orders of the agricultural population – the labourer and cottier classes – were most severely affected by the experience, though the small farmers also suffered.

The response of the British government to the famine crisis was immediate and active but, in the long run, far from adequate. Relief measures fell into four more or less distinct phases. The first was Sir Robert Peel's energetic and effective emergency provisions in 1845–6. The second consisted largely of Lord John Russell's ill-advised public works programmes in 1846–7. When these manifestly failed, Russell shifted in early 1847 to direct outdoor relief in the form of soup kitchens. The final phase, lasting from the autumn of 1847 to 1852, saw the whole relief effort placed under the authority of the Irish Poor Law Commission.[8]

Assuming the burden of responsibility for overall control of famine relief necessitated a major restructuring of the poor law administrative apparatus in Ireland. As it turned out, the English Poor Law Commission itself was deemed to need reorganisation at the same time. Consequently, both offices were rearranged in the summer of 1847. For Ireland the change marked a clear improvement in status. The old 1838 arrangement whereby Irish affairs

5 Ruth Dudley Edwards, An atlas of Irish history, London 1973, 221.
6 O' Tuathaigh, Ireland before the famine, 204.
7 Edwards, Atlas of Irish history, 221.
8 T. P. O'Neill, 'The organisation and administration of relief, 1845–52', in Dudley Edwards and Williams, Great famine: studies, 210–23.

were handled through a branch office of the English Poor Law Commission was abandoned and a separate and independent Irish Poor Law Commission was established.

The new agency was formally created by the Poor Relief (Ireland) Amendment Act of 1847 (10–11 Vic., c. 90) and consisted of the chief secretary and the under-secretary for Ireland, the former head of the Irish branch of the old commission, Edward Twisleton, who was made chief commissioner, and an assistant commissioner, Alfred Power, who, like Twisleton, was a professional poor law man.[9] The new act also provided that for the first time all destitute persons had a claim to relief, something which had not been specified in the 1838 act. Since the soup kitchen act was terminated when the new commission took up its duties, the entire responsibility for providing for famine relief as well as for the traditional poor devolved upon it and the poor law machinery. The extraordinary situation created by the famine meant that ordinary poor law procedures and rules had to be set aside for the duration of the emergency. Outdoor relief for the able-bodied, ordinarily held to a tiny percentage of total relief, had to be provided on a massive scale.

Though the 1847 potato crop was not significantly affected by the blight, the yield was small and disastrous shortages of food continued. The crop failed again in 1848 and by the summer of 1849 the Irish Poor Law Commission was still providing relief for more than a million persons, three-quarters of whom were maintained by outdoor relief.[10] Thereafter the emergency subsided. In 1850 the average daily number of persons receiving outdoor relief numbered 103,676. By 1851 it had declined to 8,559.[11]

Although the winter of 1846–7 had seen such extreme shortages of food that large numbers of people actually starved to death, it was not starvation that claimed the bulk of the lives lost during the whole of the famine period. Food stocks had been replenished by the summer of 1847 and, while scarcity continued for some years thereafter, complete failure of the food supplies was never again a critical matter. But people continued to die in large numbers, the victims of diseases which attacked the thousands weakened by malnutrition.

Fever, the inevitable companion of famine, long endemic in Ireland, reached epidemic proportions in 1846. Typhus and relapsing fever, the most prevalent forms, started sporadically and spread in an irregular fashion across the island during the following year. In Kilkenny fever cases were present in serious numbers as early as the summer of 1845, but the disease did not make its appearance in Cork until the following year.[12] Galway experienced it in the spring of 1846 while disease became widespread in Sligo and Roscommon as

---

9 Evidence relating to Ireland, *Royal Commission report*, appendices, vol. x. 17–18.
10 Ibid. 19
11 Ibid. 20.
12 MacArthur, 'Medical history of the famine', 272–3.

well as throughout Ulster in the winter of 1846-7. Most of the eastern counties escaped until 1847.

Typhus and relapsing fever were carried by lice and contagion required close contact between persons who were infested and those who were not. The famine contributed to the spread of disease because it encouraged movement of desperate people in search of food and work. Crowds of migrants moving from the poorer regions of the kingdom to the more affluent gave the epidemic the name 'road fever'.[13] This accounted for the delayed but inevitable movement of the diseases from west to east in the course of 1846 and 1847. In December 1848 the catastrophe was intensified by the appearance of cholera which had broken out in England and Scotland earlier. Cholera was independent of the famine fevers, being communicated almost entirely by contaminated water. But if not related to the famine it did prosper under the terrible conditions then characteristic of Ireland, and it added its share of misery and death to the nation's burdens.

The famine epidemic created a massive medical relief problem. The old ramshackle medical charities system, already suffering declining subscriptions prior to 1845, was quite overwhelmed by the disaster. Since it was the policy of the Russell government to make the Irish landlords assume the financial burden of famine relief both the public works scheme and poor law expenditures were to be borne by the Irish ratepayers.[14] The increase in local taxation occasioned by this approach placed an unprecedented strain on that class. Many unions were unable to cope with it and in the years 1847-9 the Irish Poor Law Commission found it necessary to dissolve no fewer than thirty boards of guardians and to appoint stipendiary guardians in their place.[15] Furthermore, since the poor rates were inadequate to meet the cost of the emergency, even when they could be collected, the government thought it necessary to impose special additional taxes. A rate-in-aid of 6d. on the pound was levied in June 1849 and another of 2d. on the pound in December 1850. These two special taxes brought in a total of £421,990 which was applied to the cost of famine relief. Thus the burden of taxation borne by the upper and middle classes in Ireland was vastly increased and the inevitable result was to reduce dramatically the amounts they customarily gave to the medical charities.

The heaviest loss was absorbed by the dispensaries and fever hospitals. In 1849 Denis Phelan, who had been reappointed to the Poor Law Commission as an inspector in 1847, toured the island investigating the effect of the famine emergency on the provision of medical care in the workhouses and medical charities.[16] He found that subscriptions for dispensaries were down

[13] Ibid.
[14] Prest, *Lord John Russell*, 269.
[15] *Royal Commission report*, 19.
[16] *Fifteenth report of the select committee of the House of Commons on the poor laws (Ireland)* (HC 1849, xv), pt II, 256.

anywhere from one-third to two-thirds, depending on the area. But worse, the district fever hospitals had been virtually wiped out. He thought not half-a-dozen were left of those traditionally supported by subscriptions and county grants. The offical returns for that year show that Phelan was close to the mark. Fever hospitals received a total of £13,000 in 1849 of which a little less than £2,000 was derived from subscriptions.[17] In 1839 fever hospital subscriptions had amounted to over £7,000. The dispensaries were somewhat better off but their subscriptions were down significantly as well, from £35,000 in 1839 to £26,000 ten years later.[18]

Not only did the famine undercut the medical charities financially, but the sheer numbers of fever victims overwhelmed the institutions physically. Facilities were clogged with suffering humanity and hundreds more clamoured to get in. Little enough could be done for the poor wretches under the best of conditions, but during the worst phases of the epidemic the situation went completely out of control in some districts.

Furthermore, the problem of treating these people was compounded by heavy mortality among the medical officers themselves. Such a fate had always been the lot of these men. William Stokes estimated that among Irish dispensary doctors in the first half of the nineteenth century about 24 per cent died in the course of their duties, more than twice the figure for military officers in combat in that period. He went on to observe in 1843 that 'Such a number of my pupils have been cut off by typhus fever as to make me feel uneasy when any of them take a dispensary office in Ireland. I look upon it almost as going into battle.'[19] In the great famine losses were especially high. In Munster forty-eight doctors died of fever alone.[20] Seven died in Cavan and eleven in Galway. Of the 473 doctors assigned by the board of health to fever duty, thirty-six were lost.

The scale of emergency created by the famine, combined with the breakdown of the medical charities, provided vastly increased scope for poor law medical care. Even before the famine the poor law authority had begun to expand its role in that area of activity. Each workhouse had an infirmary attached and employed a medical officer to look after the inmates. The 1843 select committee report revealed such inadequacies in fever hospital facilities and care that the Poor Law Commission was given statutory authority to allow boards of guardians to transport fever cases from workhouses to local fever hospitals or, if none were close by, to rent houses and convert them to such use themselves, all costs to be defrayed out of the rates.[21] Many unions took advantage of this provision.

With the advent of the famine the role of the commission increased

[17] *Abstract of returns . . . 1849*, 455.
[18] Ibid.
[19] William Stokes, *William Stokes, his life and work, 1804–78*, London 1898, 113.
[20] MacArthur, 'Medical history of the famine', 281.
[21] 'Medical charities', CSO/OP, 1846/156, 5–6.

further. In March 1846 the government passed the first of three temporary fever acts. This measure (9 Vic., c. 6) was intended to co-ordinate local relief efforts and concentrate national resources in those regions most affected by disease.[22] It empowered the lord lieutenant to appoint a temporary central board of health and to hire medical officers to serve in the most stricken counties. The board of health was duly created and consisted of Sir Randolph Routh, an army commissary officer in charge of the distribution of government food and other supplies; Edward Twistleton, the chief poor law commissioner; and three prominent Dublin physicians, Sir Robert Kane, who had served on the Playfair Commission the previous autumn, Sir Philip Crampton and Dominic Corrigan, all of whom served without pay.[23] This body had the power to compel boards of guardians to establish fever hospitals and dispensaries and to provide food, medicine and bedding for patients housed in them if local relief committees requested such intervention. All expenses incurred in establishing and maintaining these fever hospitals were to be met initially through loans from the imperial treasury, but were ultimately to be paid back out of county presentments.

While this act looked adequate on paper it worked poorly in practice. Basing the cost on county presentments, for example, required too few people to bear the burden and thus discouraged implementation.[24] Indeed, altogether too much reliance was placed on local initiative. Very few requests for intervention were received by the Central Board of Health in spite of growing need. In addition, the medical profession was much agitated by the board's composition. Kane could barely be considered a doctor any longer having virtually given up practice, and Crampton, though very eminent, was also very old. The board was actually dominated by Corrigan, a Catholic, who had made many enemies in the profession. Finally and probably because so few requests were made, the board misread the condition of the country, decided no large-scale epidemic was likely in the summer of 1846, and dissolved itself.[25] Consequently, when fever hit hard the following winter the central government was unprepared to deal with it.

In the face of the new emergency the lord lieutenant reappointed the Central Board of Health in February 1847 and it continued in being until the summer of 1850. A second fever act (10 Vic., c. 22) was passed in April 1847 and was thought to be an improvement over the first. It gave primary authority for providing medical care to the newly created relief commission and the local relief committees. Costs were to be borne by treasury advances and eventually repaid out of the poor rates. A great deal was accomplished under

---

[22] MacArthur, 'Medical history of the famine', 289.
[23] Ibid. 290. See also the account by Peter Froggatt, 'The response of the medical profession to the great famine', in E. Margaret Crawford (ed.), Famine: the Irish experience, 900–1900, Edinburgh 1989, 140–4.
[24] MacArthur, 'Medical history of the famine', 297.
[25] Froggatt, 'Response of the medical profession', 141–2.

this act but it too was unsatisfactory in many ways. The most serious short-coming in its operation, like that of its predecessor, was diffusion of authority. Conflicts between local relief committees and either the national relief commission or the Central Board of Health broke out repeatedly.[26] The Central Board found local committees very hard to budge largely because it had only an advisory role and no authority to enforce or even superintend its recommendations. There was no fixed or standard level of expenditure and the amounts spent on relief varied considerably from place to place. Great inequities occurred as a result which, when publicised, led to quarrels and recriminations among the various authorities concerned. The crux of the problem was that no single central authority had the power to control local agencies and to ensure a fair and efficient application of medical relief. Consequently, by the spring of 1848 medical relief for the poor in Ireland was deplorable and getting worse. The old medical charities system was breaking down, the temporary fever acts were not working well and were, in any event, scheduled to expire in August, and the country was in the grip of the worst fever epidemic it had ever known.

In response to this gloomy picture, Sir William Somerville, the chief secretary, drafted a bill for the better regulation of the medical charities.[27] The bill was never printed and no copy of it exists in the archives so its details are a mystery. But Somerville sent it to Sir Charles Trevelyan, the permanent under-secretary to the Treasury and a key figure in the Russell government insofar as famine relief policy was concerned, for his opinion and its broad outlines can be inferred from their correspondence. Somerville proposed establishing a central medical board with a staff of inspectors all paid out of the consolidated fund.[28] He was aware of the opposition of the medical profession to any direct link with the Poor Law Commission, so he further proposed to retain the system of financing the medical charities through the grand jury presentments.[29] Finally, given the depressed state of their finances, he also wanted government loans for the construction of fever hospitals, dispensaries and infirmaries.

Trevelyan was not pleased with these suggestions. By this time he was thoroughly sick of the Irish problem. He had involved himself in famine relief efforts to an extraordinary degree and with commendable vigour. But the recurring crop failures, the enormous amounts of money already allocated from the Treasury, and the endless conflicting reports as to the nature and extent of the emergency all combined with his strong Puritan prejudices and his suspicion of the Irish character to harden him against what he conceived

---

[26] MacArthur, 'Medical history of the famine', 297.

[27] Sir William Meredyth Somerville (1802–73), Baron Athlumney, chief secretary 1847–52, but without a seat in the Cabinet. He was much respected in Ireland for his liberal manner of running his estate.

[28] Trevelyan to Somerville, 27 May 1848, CSO/OP, 1848/351,

[29] Somerville to Trevelyan, 6 June 1848, ibid.

to be further exorbitant and unnecessary expenditures. Furthermore, he and Sir Charles Wood, the Chancellor of the Exchequer, were having great difficulty with the budget.[30] Revenue was down and cuts rather than increased spending were the order of the day.

Trevelyan rejected the proposed bill. In one long, rambling sentence he revealed the depth of his feelings on the consequences of government intervention and subsidy:

> Lavish expenditure, a slovenly wholesale way of doing business without any proper reference to local circumstances, a constant irritation between the government and the people arising from the government being placed in the relation of creditor to the great body of the people and from a natural discontent on the part of the people at their business not being done for them in the way they like, and habitual feeling of dependence and the absence of business habits on the part of those who ought to do the local business of each district, are some of the bitter fruits of this system, and my objection to your Bill is that it would perpetuate and extend the domination of this system by firmly establishing it in another large department of the social business of the country.[31]

Somerville was not put off. He himself felt deeply on the matter and was keenly aware of his responsibility to do something to alleviate the current distressed state of the country. He wrote to Trevelyan again, defending the bill, and asking the Treasury to reconsider. Trevelyan replied, again in the negative, this time justifying his position with the opinions of two obscure Treasury employees, Messrs Kennedy and Chalmers, who were attached to the paymaster's office in Dublin. In Trevelyan's view their views clinched the case in his favour. At this rejection, which indeed proved conclusive, Somerville gave expression to his frustration and rage. In a long and bitter letter he maintained that nothing Trevelyan had said induced him to alter his view as to the need for immediate legislation on this matter. The medical charities were in no condition to meet a winter of pestilence, famine and 'perhaps of Cholera', in their present condition.[32] He then went on to comment on Trevelyan's choice of advisors. Insisting that he had great regard for Mr Kennedy, Somerville none the less insisted that it had never occurred to him to consult Kennedy upon the subject of the medical charities:

> Why should I? He is kind enough to say that my observations are well deserving of consideration, but he still advises that they should be put aside. . . . As Chief Secretary for Ireland I beg to offer my protest against this system of conducting Irish business. What can Mr. Kennedy know of the Medical Charities of Ireland – how can he have acquired his knowledge? Look at his

---

[30] Prest, *Lord John Russell*, 356.

[31] Trevelyan to Somerville, 27 May 1848, CSO/OP, 1848/351.

[32] Somerville to Trevelyan, 21 June 1848, Trevelyan papers, PRO, Treasury papers, T64, 368A.

own observations upon this very Bill, and it will abundantly appear that he is to say the least, exceedingly ill-informed. . . . But what shall I say of Mr. Chalmer's letter. . . . He seems half ashamed of the task imposed upon him, for he begins by saying that he considers himself unable to form any just opinion as to the workings of the Bill, and in this I quite agree with him – but . . . he winds up by giving it as his opinion that H. E. [Clarendon] should be allowed time to make up his mind upon so important a subject. Now I put it to yourself as a Gentleman acquainted with Office – is it not too bad to see the affairs of a great country thus administered – that a Bill upon which much pains have been bestowed, that has been submitted to the Lord Lieutenant over and over again, . . . – that deals with no less a question than the Medical treatment of the sick poor of the most afflicted country in the universe, should be thus referred to a Scotch clerk in Mr. Kennedy's office whose experience of Ireland is probably confined to a lounge in Sackville Street, or a trip per railway to Kingstown – I repeat that it is too bad, I had almost said humiliating.[33]

'Treasury control' was a spectre which haunted many tales of Victorian administration. The fate of the 1848 Medical Charities Bill is one of the better examples.

Though unwilling to consider a comprehensive reform of the medical charities, the government nevertheless had to do something. Their solution was a third temporary fever act passed in September dealing with the problem of inadequate centralised control of medical relief by concentrating authority in the Poor Law Commission.[34] The Central Board of Health was renewed. But the appointment of medical officers, the power to fix salaries and the management of all temporary fever hospitals and dispensaries, whether established under the first two fever acts or the third, were transferred to the boards of guardians. The poor law commissioners were given extensive powers to oversee and direct the guardians in their efforts. Furthermore, the appearance of cholera produced a further centralising measure, the Nuisances Removal and Diseases Prevention Act of 1848 (11/12 Vic., c. 123), often called the Cholera Act. It gave the lord lieutenant (and the Central Board of Health, while that body continued to exist) the power to place any area of the country under the authority of the act which then required the guardians to clean streets and public places, remove nuisances (by which the Victorians meant accumulations of filth), bury the dead, and provide medical facilities, medicines and care for persons in need.[35] Thus the poor law apparatus was increasingly involved in public health and medical care activities. Upon the final dissolution of the Central Board of Health in 1850 its role in administering the new act was taken over by the Irish Poor Law Commission.

The temporary fever acts expired in August 1850. They had not prevented

---

33 Ibid.
34 Medicus, *Observations*, 33.
35 Ibid. 37.

great loss of life; but Woodham-Smith, who is far from being an enthusiast for British policy in these years, feels that on the whole they were a success.[36] Much good and useful sanitary work had been done and fever hospital and dispensary accommodation for 23,000 patients had been created at a cost of £119,000. From July 1847 (when weekly returns began to be kept regularly) to August 1850, almost 600,000 persons had been treated in government dispensaries and hospitals.[37] Recently scholars have taken to arguing that the Irish Poor Law Commission was party to a policy of restricted relief aimed at driving the cottiers off their land so as to facilitate consolidation.[38] Whatever London and the Treasury Lords may have had in mind, it appears, none the less, that the Poor Law Commission and its servants on the various adminis-trative levels involved were sensitive to the terrible problems to be faced and earned much respect in the way they carried out their duties. McDowell states that they demonstrated energy, courage, efficiency and devotion to their duty in these years.[39] While they were still faced with much traditional hostility among the population and the medical community, their claim to the administration of the whole medical charities system was greatly strengthened by their performance. Moreover, it was clear to some observers that the role of the poor law authority was bound to increase because even allowing for the dissolution of many of the improvised facilities in the wake of the emergency, there was a substantial and permanent increase in the number of poor-law fever hospitals.

In March 1850 Somerville at last introduced a medical charities bill in the Commons.[40] It provided for a central board to be composed of the two poor law commissioners, the chief secretary, the under secretary and two or three distinguished medical men to be appointed by the lord lieutenant. This body was to be known as the Commission of Health and was to have an office staff, secretary and four inspectors. The dispensaries, fever hospitals and county infirmaries were to come under its jurisdiction and were to be financed through the poor rate. The Commission was to have the power to create dispensary and hospital districts and to rationalise and reorganise the entire medical relief system. Committees composed of poor law guardians and rate-payers selected by the guardians were to manage on the local level.

Emotions ran high among the Irish doctors. This appeared to be the end for the old dispensary system. Uncertainty had hung over it for years and in its weakened financial condition all agreed something had to be done. The

---

36 Cecil Woodham–Smith, *The great hunger*, London 1962, 197.

37 MacArthur, 'Medical history of the famine', 298.

38 Christine Kinealy, 'The poor law during the great famine', in Crawford, *Famine*, 157–75. See also James S. Donnelly, Jr, 'The administration of relief, 1847–51', in Vaughn, *Ireland under the union*, I: *1801–70*, 316–31.

39 McDowell, *Irish administration*, 182–3.

40 *Bill for the better distribution, support and management of the medical charities in Ireland* (HC 1850, iv), 27–40.

Dublin Medical Press was cautious in its appraisal but concluded that while a clause here or there would have to be changed, it could support the new measure as a whole.[41] Petitions and letters poured in from all parts of the kingdom, most supporting the bill.[42] The only negative note within the profession was sounded by the county infirmary surgeons. The *DMP* was sympathetic, arguing that there should be special provision to safeguard their prescriptive, corporate rights.

The bill had a difficult passage. As always with all but the most vital measures, Irish legislation was frequently postponed and taken up late in the evening, usually before a thin house. Other business seemed to be forever taking priority. The *DMP* hung on every debate and was easily exasperated by this practice. On 3 July, in reference to the Don Pacifico affair, Jacob commented tartly, 'Parliament has been so busy providing for the political charities of Greece that it has had no time to deal with the medical charities of Ireland.'[43]

Somerville too found the task of appeasing all interested parties increasingly difficult. The key problem became the composition of the central board. The medical interest wanted three members, two of whom would be unpaid. These would be in reality honorary positions to be occupied by two of the Dublin greats who would think it beneath their dignity (and professionally too confining) to accept a paid position. The poor law commissioner (now Alfred Power who succeeded Twistleton upon his resignation in 1849), on the other hand, wanted a single, paid, medical commissioner. A strong case could be made against unpaid commissioners on any kind of board: they might devote insufficient time to the commission, they might be susceptible to bribes or other forms of influence, very likely they would be hard to control. Power was concerned with these potential problems. He apparently feared the effect of too many difficult Irish doctors on a commission which was to administer a large, sprawling, medical care system. Very likely he felt that as long as the money came from the poor rate and he was the poor law commissioner then he should have the clear upper hand. Somerville's correspondence with Clarendon on this point in both 1850 and 1851 stresses Power's resistence to strong medical influence on the board, either in the form of too many doctors or in the persons of particularly difficult doctors such as Dominic John Corrigan, a noted maverick. It is also clear from this correspondence that both Somerville and Clarendon thought highly of Power and were unwilling to weaken his position in any way.[44]

---

41 *DMP* xxiii (1850), 237–8.

42 Correspondence with the chief secretary on the Medical Charities Bill, CSO/OP, 1850/18.

43 *DMP* xxiv (1850), 15.

44 Somerville to Clarendon, 28 May 1850, Clarendon papers, Oxford, Bodleian Library, Deposit Irish, box 28. George William Frederick Villiers (1800–70), 4th earl of Clarendon and 4th Baron Hyde, entered the diplomatic service when still virtually a boy. In 1823 he

Until it was manifestly impossible Somerville fought for three medical commissioners. Such an arrangement would provide positions for the important Dublin doctors he wanted to reward, and would make it less likely that the medical profession could accuse him of throwing them to the poor law commissioners. On the other hand, it is equally clear that he did not want the doctors to dominate the board.[45] Hence he favoured a rather large commission totalling seven members – the chief secretary, the under-secretary, the two poor law commissioners and three medical men. The problem lay in the attitude of the House of Commons which insisted that a five-member board would be better.[46]

The two honorary medical commissionerships would probably have been dropped in any event, but at this point a completely unrelated administrative question intervened to clinch the matter. For some time the Russell government had been considering eliminating the office of lord lieutenant and placing Irish affairs in the hands of a fourth secretary of state. For reasons we need not go into here this led to reorganisation in a number of Irish departments including the Poor Law Commission which was to receive an additional commissioner. Power favoured filling the new post with a medical man. Somerville put the problem this raised to Clarendon quite succinctly: 'The difficulty of this proposal seems to be that you cannot have two boards, at least I think so, composed of equally the same members – It would be fairly asked why not combine them? And then I suppose we should have the medical profession up in arms.'[47] Beyond the question of composition Somerville faced another difficulty which he described as the 'cantankerous disposition of the Irish M.P.s'. Any Irish legislation was made 'arduous' by their increasing tendency to carp and criticise for what he took to be their own amusement.[48]

The bill was read for the first time on 26 March 1850 but did not get serious consideration until 12 July.[49] Somerville's fears that the composition of the board would be attacked were borne out. But all major amendments

was appointed commissioner of customs and became well acquainted with Irish affairs at this time. In the mid-thirties he performed a delicate diplomatic mission to the court of Spain with such tact and skill that his reputation among the politically influential was established. A Whig, he entered the Melbourne government in 1840 when it was in great difficulty. He returned to office with the Whigs in 1846 and was made lord lieutenant the following year, a post which he held until 1852 under extremely trying circumstances. By the mid-nineteenth century the position of lord lieutenant was usually held by a wealthy nonentity, while political influence was coming to reside with the chief secretary. Clarendon was an exception to this trend. He rather than Somerville carried real political weight, a fact which their correspondence makes clear: DNB xx. 347–50.

45 Somerville to Clarendon, 28 May 1850, Clarendon papers, box 28.
46 Somerville to Clarendon, 16 May 1850, ibid.
47 Somerville to Clarendon, 28 May 1850, ibid.
48 Somerville to Clarendon, 21 April 1850, ibid.
49 Hansard, cxii. (1850), 1289–91.

were beaten down in four difficult sessions in late July and early August.[50] By this time the bill had been postponed so many times that the *Dublin Medical Press* had about given it up. Then suddenly, on 10 August, it reached the Lords where, after a momentary flurry of excitement, it died, their lordships insisting they had not time to consider so important a measure. However, some of those who voted to drop it expressed the hope that a similar bill would be submitted the following year.[51]

The sources reveal little about what happened. Somerville's correspondence with Clarendon is full of medical charities news in April and May but contains nothing for the July–August period when debate was most intense. His letters in the spring suggest that he was having great difficulty lining up the votes he needed. He complained that the Commons was not 'manageable' and that the Irish members were particularly difficult. Faced with these conditions he may have tried to finesse the bill through a thin house at the end of the session and got caught when his opponents moved quickly enough to urge the Lords to shelve it. Evidence of a kind exists for this view. On 3 February 1851 a letter appeared in the *DMP* from a Dr E. G. Brunker, surgeon at the Louth County Infirmary at Dundalk.[52] Basically it was a complaint that a recent meeting at the College of Surgeons in Dublin had been packed with supporters of Somerville's bill. However, as if to demonstrate the power of the bill's opponents, Bunker went to some length to explain why it had failed in the previous parliamentary session. He had been in London in the spring of 1850 representing a group of infirmary surgeons who were attempting to persuade Somerville to drop the infirmaries from the proposed measure. They met twice in April and clearly did not get on for Somerville wrote to Clarendon on 21 April that

> When I undertook the Medical Charities Bill I knew that the subject was a dangerous one and that it would give me great trouble – but I believe that of all the Bills come before Parliament it will be the most beneficial and therefore I shall do everything in my power to carry it. I am not at all frightened by the opposition of the Infirmary doctors. I will do all I can to protect their just rights – but I owe thirty-two gentlemen must not be permitted to prevent the social improvement of the country.[53]

Bunker hinted that the delay in bringing the bill forward was premeditated. He observed that when the key debates were held in late July and early August, many Irish members were absent because they had assumed it would not come up again. If these men had been present Bunker was confident they would have forced amendments preserving the infirmaries from the effects of the bill. As it was, he maintained, the bill had passed the Commons in 'a very

[50] Ibid. cxiii (1850), 146, 221, 888–91, 951.
[51] Ibid. 1012.
[52] *DMP* xxv (1851), 94.
[53] Somerville to Clarendon, 21 April 1850, Clarendon papers, box 28.

thin house' and it had been his, Bunker's, intervention with 'a noble Lord' which had resulted in its demise in the Lords. Speaking in the final debate in the Lords on 12 August Lord Redesdale also seemed to suggest that the government had been caught in a manoeuvre. He maintained that responsibility for postponement of the bill had rested with the government 'who had impeded and delayed its progress in the House of Commons'.[54]

Throughout the winter of 1850–1 Irish medical circles were thick with rumours about yet another medical charities bill. In January a massive meeting of dispensary and fever hospital medical officers was held at the College of Surgeons in St Stephens Green. Opinion was heavily in favour of government action. A monster petition was got up supporting the chief secretary's efforts in securing aid for their beleaguered institutions.[55]

Somerville responded with a new bill significantly different from its predecessor. The separate medical board, which had generated so much debate the previous session, had been dropped to be replaced by a reorganised Poor Law Commission which was to include a medical commissioner.[56] Somerville explained that the new formula had grown out of discussions he had had with various MPs and that this was their preference.[57] The *Dublin Medical Press*, which had usually supported Somerville's efforts, momentarily gave vent to its real position. 'Never within our memory . . . has our profession in Ireland been placed in greater peril', began an editorial of 19 March. It went on to trace the sad history of attempts at medical charities legislation and concluded that 'plainly . . . the medical profession has no trustworthy representative just now in Dublin Castle'.[58] But this was only a flash of temper, an expression of accumulated frustration. Alexander Knox, a rising young surgeon who had been secretary to the acting committee of medical attendants to dispensaries and fever hospitals, formed at the January meeting in the College of Surgeons which had triggered Bunker's letter, responded with a spirited defence of Somerville and the virtues of the new bill.[59] The *DMP* soon came around to reality as well. Upon reconsideration it concluded that the proposed medical commissionership seemed to be vested with real power and that all depended upon the calibre of the man who would fill the position. In all other respects the new bill differed little from its predecessor.[60]

Throughout the spring the Irish doctors met and discussed and petitioned for or against the impending bill. The overwhelming majority of the letters and petitions that poured into the chief secretary's office and to the *Dublin*

---

54 *Hansard*, cxiii (1850), 1012.
55 *DMP* xxv (1851), 38–44.
56 *Bill for the better distribution, support and management of the medical charities in Ireland* (HC 1851, iv), 169–71.
57 *Hansard*, cxv (1851), 899.
58 *DMP* xxv (1851), 190.
59 Ibid. 206.
60 Ibid. 221.

Medical Press favoured the measure.[61] There was one important exception, however. The infirmary surgeons had formed their own society in the previous year and they pressed hard for exclusion from the proposed change.[62]

As in the previous year Somerville found it difficult to make progress in the Commons. The bill was read a second time in early April but serious debate in committee did not begin until 25 June. However this time the problem was not merely the traditional tendency to postpone non-critical Irish legislation. Everything was delayed in the spring of 1851 owing to the endless wrangling over the Ecclesiastical Titles Bill, the government's reaction to the pope's announcement the previous year of his intention to establish a regular episcopal hierarchy in Great Britain. The bill sought to make illegal the assumption of titles by Catholic prelates taken from any place name in the British Isles. Lord John Russell assumed the leadership of outraged Protestantism, and debate on this very emotional issue went on from February until the end of June. In spite of much advice to the contrary, Lord John had insisted on including Ireland in the bill. Consequently, he encountered vigorous resistance from Irish members in the Commons.[63] There was no way the Irish members could hope to stop the bill, for it received sizable majorities at every stage of its progress, but they could harass the government with prolonged debate and obstruct every other measure the government brought forward.[64]

These circumstances placed Somerville in an impossible position. He complained to Clarendon throughout the spring. On 9 May he wrote, 'I dread the renewal of the Papal Debate. We had another scene in the House last night . . . I am very sorry that I cannot get in my Irish Bills – I have about eight of them now of great importance to the country.'[65] On 20 June he saw a glimmer of hope. 'The House is once more in Committee on the Ecclesiastical Titles Bill and there seems on the part of the Irish Brigade [the militant core of the nationalist party] to be a disposition not to talk so much.'[66] A few days later he felt it was all over. 'The Brigade appears to have exhausted all of their powder.'[67]

But the effect of this experience was to force Somerville to defend all his measures in the last month or two of the session. Even after the Ecclesiastical Titles Bill had passed, the Irish members remained sullen and unco-operative. He complained on 17 July that 'the disposition of the Irish members seems to be to allow nothing to pass'.[68]

---

61 CSO/OP, 1851/47 contains a large collection of letters and petitions to the chief secretary regarding the Medical Charities Bill.
62 *DMP* xxv (1851), 237–8.
63 Ibid.
64 J. H. Whyte, *The Independent Irish party, 1850–59*, London 1958, 21.
65 Somerville to Clarendon, 9 May 1851, Clarendon papers, box 28.
66 Somerville to Clarendon, 20 June 1851, ibid.
67 Somerville to Clarendon, 28 June 1851, ibid.
68 Somerville to Clarendon, 17 July 1851, ibid.

The Medical Charities Bill entered the committee stage on 25 June. Few members objected to its principles but there was much debate on the details of funding and management. Most important, some members continued to resist Somerville's inclusion of the infirmaries and fever hospitals.[69] Worn down by the entire two years' effort, the chief secretary capitulated to his strongest and most persistent opponents and agreed to exclude the county infirmaries from the scope of the bill. 'As I may be said to live now in the House of Commons, I fear I may not be able to see you before I go down to that time wasting assembly tomorrow', he bitterly observed to Clarendon on 27 July. He then went on to explain his decision:

> I have gone through the Dispensary Clauses on the Medical Charities Bill – and despairing of carrying the measure in its complete form, and alive to the responsibility of leaving the present Dispensary establishment to perish, thus depriving the poor of all Medical relief, I mean, if you see no objection, to confine the Bill for the present session to Dispensaries. I shall thus have laid the foundation for a more complete measure hereafter – though nothing but my conviction that I can do no more would lead me to this omission – which I have frequently declared I would not make – I feel however that of the two responsibilities this is the least.[70]

Somerville tried to retain inclusion of the fever hospitals but this too failed; and when the bill passed on 1 August it applied to the dispensaries only. After fifteen years of debate, conflict and anxious effort, the Irish dispensaries had obtained a measure of security and centralisation. In the autumn of 1851 the medical profession in Ireland awaited the first moves of the poor law commissioners.

69 *Hansard*, cxvii (1851), 1244.
70 Somerville to Clarendon, 27 July 1851, Clarendon papers, box 28.

5

The Medical Charities Act and the Development of Poor Law Medical Relief in Ireland, 1851–1875

The Medical Charities (Ireland) Act (14 & 15 Vic., c. 68) marked a far more significant shift in the nature of poor relief in Ireland than has generally been recognised. It is usually referred to as the Dispensary Act because it brought the dispensaries under the jurisdiction of the Irish Poor Law Commission. Certainly it did that. But historians have failed to appreciate the effect of the new medical relief responsibilities upon the poor law authority or the broader public health powers contained in the act. Specifically the new measure accomplished three things: it turned the beleaguered dispensary system over to the Irish Poor Law Commission; it reorganised that agency by requiring it to have a medical commissioner and medical inspectors; and, by giving the commission the authority to enforce the Nuisances Removal and Diseases Prevention Acts of 1848 and 1849 in periods when the country was threatened by epidemic disease, it transformed the commission into something like a national board of health. The Medical Charities Act, therefore, concentrated in the Irish Poor Law Commission medical relief and public health powers unprecedented in Ireland and unparalleled in the rest of the United Kingdom until the creation of the English Local Government Board in 1871.

It will be recalled that the Irish Poor Law Commission had been reorganised as recently as 1847 when separated from its English parent organisation and consisted on the top level of two ex-officio members, the chief and under-secretaries, and two permanent members, the chief and assistant poor law commissioners. The Medical Charities Act changed this arrangement by adding a medical commissioner and abolishing the post of assistant commissioner, replacing it with another full poor law commissioner so as to ensure that in the absence of the chief commissioner administrative control of the commission would devolve on a poor law officer rather than on the medical commissioner who, it was thought, would be unlikely to have appropriate experience in general poor law matters.[1]

The Poor Law Commission was one of the largest and most powerful government departments in Ireland. In the late 1840s, its ranks swollen by the demands of the famine emergency, the commission employed no fewer

[1] *Bromley-Stephenson report*, 1.

than fifty-eight inspectors and 121 clerks.[2] But as the crisis eased in the early fifties staffing was cut back to more modest levels. The Medical Charities Act added five medical inspectors in 1851, but by the following year reductions among general poor law inspectors lowered the total inspectorate to twenty-one. In the course of the 1850s pauperism declined markedly all across Ireland and further contractions of the staff were demanded by the Treasury. By 1861 it consisted of nine poor law inspectors, four medical inspectors, four auditors and forty-one clerks.[3] None the less this remained a large establishment for a population of less than six million persons. The English Poor Law Board was not significantly larger though serving a population three times as great.

The size of the Irish commission was determined by the extraordinary powers and duties it possessed which were in turn a function of the very special circumstances characteristic of Irish government and politics at this time. The threat to traditional relationships and procedures presented by the movement for Catholic Emancipation and O'Connell's Repeal agitation had led Irish governments of the 1830s and 1840s to abandon the time-honoured policy of explicit support for the Protestant landlords in favour of a neutrality which sought to minimise sectarianism. As a result the old framework of local government, which had been controlled by the Protestant gentry, collapsed and was replaced by a centralised administration more wide-ranging and influential in the various aspects of local affairs than any other in the United Kingdom. Thomas Larcom (1801–79), the under-secretary from 1853 to 1869, put it best in an 1857 memorandum to a new chief secretary:

> Thirty years ago the problem of government in Ireland was to govern a million people who governed the other six million. When they were emancipated the problem was to govern the seven million and the local machinery having been destroyed, to do so by the direct action of the executive.[4]

The authority of the Irish Poor Law Commission reflected this situation. It possessed power over taxation, poor law property, the supervision of guardians' conduct and even the existence of their boards, not shared by its English counterpart.

For example, in England the unit of taxation for the poor law system was

---

2 *Fourteenth and ninth annual report of the poor law commissioners under the Poor Relief (Ireland) Act and the Medical Charities (Ireland) Act* (HC 1861, xxviii), 333. The first report of the Irish Poor Law Commission under the provisions of the Medical Charities Act appeared in February 1853. From 1853 through 1859 the commission reported on its medical charities activity and its routine activity separately. From 1860 onward the reports were combined, hence the curious title.

3 Ibid. 334. By way of comparison, the staff of the English Poor Law Board consisted of 13 inspectors and 43 clerks: Treasury minute of 12 Dec. 1866, PRO, Treasury papers, T. 1/6650A/17927.

4 Thomas Larcom to Lord Naas, memorandum of July 1857, Mayo papers, Dublin, National Library of Ireland, MS 11190.

the parish, which for poor law purposes was unique and unchangeable, while in Ireland the unit of taxation was the electoral division, which consisted of a number of ancient Irish territorial units known as townlands.[5] Electoral divisions had been created by the poor law authorities in 1838 and could be enlarged or sub-divided at the will of the commission. In Ireland the building and renting of workhouses, dispensaries and other poor law facilities was done by the commission and all the property associated with them was vested in it rather than in the boards of guardians as was the case in England. Consequently, all matters pertaining to this property – maintenance, additional construction, repairs and sundry other details – required the attention and decision of the commission; that is to say, had to be handled on the central rather than local level. Religious observances required careful judgement. The commission was obliged to appoint workhouse chaplains and see to the regulation of services for the inmates, a duty demanding both delicacy and tact in a country where such matters so frequently raised angry discord among ratepayers and guardians of different creeds. In order to meet their responsibilities under the law the commissioners had to supervise the work of the guardians very closely. The minutes of each weekly meeting of each of the 163 boards of guardians had to be read and compared to the detailed evaluations contained in the inspectors' reports.[6] Other examples of the extraordinary centralisation of poor law administration in Ireland, particularly with regard to medical services, will be taken up later. But the above examples should be sufficient to make the point. Perhaps the ultimate difference in the powers of the Irish and English poor law authorities lay in the fact that only the former had the legal right to dissolve boards of guardians and replace them with officials paid to conduct union affairs. And let it not be thought that this was but a theoretical power. Under the desperate conditions imposed by the famine emergency the Irish Poor Law Commission had found it necessary to implement it no fewer than thirty-nine times.[7]

Possessing such power, and required thereby to supervise local administration of poor law business with minute care, the commission developed an intimate and, for the most part, co-operative relationship with the guardians. In the course of the two decades following the famine it rarely encountered difficulty in getting its orders carried out.[8] When differences of opinion did arise and particular boards of guardians refused to comply with the commis-

---

[5] *Bromley-Stephenson report*, 1.

[6] Ibid. 6.

[7] Ibid. Note that this authority was very like that enjoyed by the Irish administration with respect to stipendiary magistrates or, as they were commonly called in Ireland, resident magistrates.

[8] The IPLC found it necessary to invoke their power to suspend boards of guardians on only one occasion between 1851 and 1872. See the case of the guardians of Millstreet Union, County Cork, Oct. 1871–Mar.1872: *Twenty-fifth and twentieth annual report* (HC 1872, xxix), 2223.

sion's wishes, the latter resorted to the courts with invariable success. The commission's performance and record in these decades was a product of more than its legal authority, however. The way that authority was used was a critical component of its success and that, in turn, depended upon leadership. For most of the 1850s and 1860s the commission was dominated by two extremely able and energetic men who made maximum use of their positions – Alfred Power and Thomas Larcom.

Alfred Power (1805–88) was an Englishman, the youngest son of a physician.[9] He attended Cambridge on a scholarship and subsequently studied at the Middle Temple, becoming a barrister in 1830. After practising law for a few years he began his career in public service when selected by Nassau Senior, the noted economist and chairman of the investigatory poor law commission, to be an assistant commissioner in 1833. Upon the passage of the Poor Law Amendment Act (1834) Power was retained in his post in the new poor law administration. In due course he was assigned to help establish the reformed poor law system in the northern English counties, a job which tested his abilities and character to the utmost given the savage resistance encountered in that region. Edwin Chadwick, writing to Lord John Russell in 1838, noted that 'Alfred Power "has been pursued by wild persons intent on assassinating him and has three times been assaulted with serious intent".'[10]

In 1843 Power was transferred to the Irish branch of the poor law administration. Upon the resignation of Edward Twistleton, chief commissioner from 1847 to 1849, he succeeded to that post, serving until the creation of the Irish Local Government Board in 1872. Under the subsequent reorganisation he was appointed vice president of the board, the chief administrative position. Power retired in 1879. He was awarded a CB in 1871 and a KCB in 1874.[11]

Power was obviously a first-class administrator, highly valued by his political superiors. Somerville and Clarendon both pressed for his appointment as chief commissioner in 1849.[12] Many years later Lord Hartington, then chief secretary in Gladstone's first administration, in a letter to the prime minister, described Power as one of the 'ablest and most efficient public servants in Ireland' and said that he had administered the poor law 'almost from its commencement with great strictness, although, . . . with great wisdom'.[13]

---

9   *Biograph and Review* ns, pt III, 1882, 229–32.
10 Quoted in Finer, *Chadwick*, 141.
11 With reference to proposing him for the KCB, Gladstone wrote to Power in 1874, 'Sir, Upon the resignation of office, I have thought it my duty to review the list of those who may be justly regarded as the most distinguished among the many excellent and able men in the civil service of this country, with a view to the best possible use of one or two marks of honour now at my disposal': *Biograph and Review*, 232.
12 Somerville to Clarendon, 15 Mar. 1849, Clarendon papers, box 28.
13 Hartington to Gladstone, 23 Jan. 1873, Gladstone papers, BL, Add. MS 44144, fos 31–2.

A devoted disciple of the principles of 1834, Power was an outspoken adherent of the concept of maximum indoor relief. No region of the British Isles devoted a higher proportion of its expenditure on the poor to that form of relief than Ireland in the 1850s and 1860s. Power came in for a great deal of criticism as a result of this policy but it should be borne in mind that he alone was not responsible for it. The statute which defined the administrative structure and legal powers of the Irish Poor Law Commission said nothing about what form relief should take. The proportion of indoor to outdoor relief was a policy decision which changed from time to time and involved the guardians as much or more than the central authority. Power could only hope to persuade for he could not coerce the local boards on this issue. When many of them moved toward greater emphasis on outdoor relief in the late 1860s Power went along with them although he disapproved.

Power's philosophical attachment to indoor relief did not mean that he failed to appreciate the advantages of large-scale medical relief outside the workhouses. On the contrary, he was equally committed to state medicine and public health. The dispensary system was expanded significantly during his tenure, workhouse infirmaries were broadened in function to allow treatment of non-paupers and paying patients, and no agency of the state anywhere in the United Kingdom demonstrated greater efficiency or built up a better record in epidemic control and vaccination than the Irish Poor Law Commission in this period. In his last years at the Local Government Board he was instrumental in drafting the Irish Public Health Acts of 1874 and 1878, which codified Irish sanitary legislation. The seriousness with which Power took public health work is revealed by the dedication to a curious little collection of children's poems he published in 1871. Entitled *Sanitary rhymes. . . . personal practices against cholera and all kinds of fever*, it was dedicated to 'the Founder of Sanitary Legislation, Edwin Chadwick, . . . by a fellow worker in the same field'.

The other important figure in the development of poor law policy in this period was Thomas Larcom (1801–79) who was the under-secretary in the Irish administration from 1853 to 1868.[14] The son of an English naval officer, he was educated at the Royal Military Academy at Woolwich and subsequently joined the Royal Engineers. Assigned to the ordnance survey he was transferred to Ireland in 1828 where he spent the rest of his life. Early in his career Larcom demonstrated leadership, initiative and wide-ranging abilities, qualities which took him rapidly to the top of Irish public administration. Assigned the task of making county surveys in the mid-thirties, he and his staff produced not only accurate, beautiful and innovative maps, but valuable compilations of historical and cultural information as well. As census commissioner in 1841 he demonstrated the same ability to expand the scope of his assignments. The Irish census of that year set the standard

[14] *DNB* xi, 584–6.

adopted in England the following decade. By 1846 he was made commissioner of public works just in time to oversee the massive relief programmes used to provide employment in the first stages of the famine. Upon his appointment as under-secretary in 1853, the post was made non-political and permanent.

Larcom was both a friend and disciple of Thomas Drummond (1797–1840), the popular reforming under-secretary of the Whig administration of 1835–41. Like Drummond he adhered closely to a policy of expanding the influence and authority of Dublin Castle in order to maintain order, reduce religious conflict and exploitation, and promote the material well-being of the entire country. As a centraliser Larcom was naturally a strong supporter of the Poor law Commission. In a typical memorandum to a lord lieutenant in 1854 Larcom explained that the new medical relief and poor law services had

> removed or are rapidly removing from our community the Ignorance which formerly pervaded the people and the inevitable sufferings of poverty and sickness, infirmity and helplessness which belong to all societies; and this relief has allowed the adult, the active and the healthy to spring forward in improvement.[15]

Even though he was primarily occupied with the details of running the Irish government, Larcom was in a position to exert a significant and continuous influence on the formulation and conduct of poor law policy. Unlike its English counterpart, the Irish Poor Law Commission actually met as a body. Twice each week the permanent commissioners met the chief secretary and the under-secretary at the latter's offices in Dublin Castle.[16] However, since the chief secretaryship was a position which changed hands with every shift in the English government and, moreover, required its incumbent to be in Westminster to defend Irish policy in the Commons for much of the year, the under-secretary, once the post became permanent, was in a position to play the more important role. For much of the two decades under consideration Larcom was intimately involved with the poor law administration.

From the point of view of the Irish medical community the key provision of the Medical Charities Act was the appointment of a medical commissioner. The legacy of distrust generated by a decade of conflict over the administration of the medical charities made the appointment especially critical. It was vital that the new commissioner be someone the medical profession respected and in whom it could have confidence. On the other hand, he had to be a person with whom the government and poor law officials could work. The requirements for the post were quite broad, the act

---

[15] Larcom to Lord St Germans, Jan. 1854, Larcom papers, Dublin, National Library of Ireland, MS 7600, no. 4.

[16] *Bromley-Stephenson report*, 4.

stating only that the medical commissioner be a physician or surgeon with at least ten years' experience.[17]

As with other such appointments the selection process was the business of top government figures – the lord lieutenant, chief secretary, and in this case, the chief poor law commissioner – and was shrouded in the usual secrecy. In the months following the passage of the act the Dublin press and the medical community buzzed with anxious rumours concerning the chances of this or that supposed candidate. Indeed, the task of finding the right man was protracted because it was initially complicated by the political debts owed by the government to certain Irish doctors who had supported it in recent years. Foremost among them was Dominic John Corrigan.

As a prominent Dublin physician with an international reputation Corrigan had unimpeachable credentials for the post. For many years he had been an outspoken supporter of the government's efforts to promote poor law control of the medical charities. One of the three medical members of the Central Board of Health during the famine, he had worked closely with leading members of the government and impressed them with his energy and administrative ability. Sir William Somerville was convinced Corrigan had first claim to the position.[18]

But Corrigan's appointment would have been very controversial. His caustic tongue and record of support for the Irish Poor Law Commission had won him many powerful enemies among medical men. The Irish College of Surgeons and the *Dublin Medical Press* had considered him a government pet ever since their quarrel over the Medical Charities Bill of 1842. Other members of the profession had been alienated by his administration of medical relief during the famine. He was accused of trying to bully the board of health and of being chiefly responsible for the paltry fee of 5s. per day paid to medical officers employed to combat the fever epidemic of 1847–9.[19] Probably none of this would have mattered very much if the government itself had found him satisfactory. But it did not. Power, who had worked with him, told Somerville he found Corrigan vain and difficult and dreaded the thought of him as a colleague.[20] A man of honour, the chief secretary felt strongly enough about his political obligations to offer Corrigan the position in spite of Power's opposition. But everyone was relieved when he refused to accept, apparently considering the salary insufficient.

With the most obvious candidate out of the running and at the suggestion of the lord lieutenant, Somerville approached Sir Philip Crampton about the position. But Crampton, an even more distinguished member of the Irish medical elite than Corrigan and much less divisive, would not even consider

[17] 14 & 15 Vic., c. 68, *Statutes at large*, v. 91, 319.
[18] Somerville to Clarendon, 12 Aug. 1851, Clarendon papers, box 28.
[19] Froggatt, 'Response of the medical profession', 144–5.
[20] Somerville to Clarendon, 12 Aug. 1851, Clarendon papers, box 28.

the post. He was very old and ill and died within two years. Good form having been observed in offering old supporters the major piece of patronage resulting from the act, a much broader range of candidates could now be canvassed. The process went on into the autumn while the dispensary medical officers awaited the announcement apprehensively. On 10 September the *Dublin Medical Press* observed that 'The great question is the appointment of the Medical Commissioner. . . . Strange to say, this valuable morsel of patronage has (we gather from good authority) been refused by two gentlemen already, and still hangs dangling from candidate to candidate like a roasted apple on the end of a string on the eve of Allhallows.' [21] Finally, after months of deliberation on the merits of several worthy but lesser known men, the government announced the appointment of Dr John M'Donnell (1796–1892), professor of anatomy at the Irish College of Surgeons.

Probably no selection could have pleased the profession more. M'Donnell's credentials were close to ideal. In a letter to Clarendon, Sir Thomas Redington, under-secretary in 1851, wrote that M'Donnell had 'a very high character . . . many friends in and out of the profession especially among the Liberal party and there is no doubt of his ability being great'.[22] Born in Belfast, the son of a locally prominent doctor, he had been educated at Trinity College and apprenticed under Richard Carmichael, the founder of the Irish Medical Association. Subsequently M'Donnell had studied in Edinburgh, Paris and London before establishing his practice in Dublin.[23] In 1827 he had been made a member of the College of Surgeons and twenty years later assumed the position of professor of anatomy there.

M'Donnell served as medical commissioner for twenty-five years. He was responsible for the supervision of medical personnel and practice in the dispensaries, fever hospitals and workhouse infirmaries and for providing medical advice to the other commissioners when the commission was responsible for implementing the various public health acts. The loss of the internal records of the Irish Poor Law Commission makes it impossible to assess his precise impact within that body but the absence of controversy within either the medical press or the correspondence of the Irish government suggests that he did a competent if unspectacular job. Certainly the selection of a respected member of the College of Surgeons did much to reduce the suspicion many members of the medical profession still felt towards the Poor Law Commission.

Yet another step required by the Medical Charities Act was the addition of medical personnel to the poor law inspectorate. Drawn from the ranks of surgeons and physicians of seven years' standing these officials, like their counterparts among the regular poor law inspectors, were each assigned terri-

21 *DMP* xxvi (1851), 174.
22 Redington to Clarendon, Oct. 1851, Clarendon papers, box 25.
23 Sir Charles A. Cameron, *A history of the Royal College of Surgeons in Ireland and of the Irish Schools of Medicine*, 2nd edn, Dublin 1916, 614–15.

tories consisting of a varying number of poor law unions within which they were responsible for the inspection of poor law medical facilities and practice. Initially the new medical inspectors were fully occupied with the reorganisation and assimilation of the dispensaries into the poor law system. Thereafter their normal duties consisted of regular circuits through their districts examining the buildings, equipment, medicines and care provided in the dispensaries, fever hospitals and workhouse infirmaries. Owing to the magnitude of the task of reorganisation five rather than the anticipated four medical inspectors were appointed in 1851. However, in 1855 the number was reduced to four and then, in 1871, to three.[24] These cutbacks were partly a function of the more or less constant Treasury pressure for economy. But they also reflected a shift in the Poor Law Commission's conception of what inspectors did and what credentials they needed to do it.

In the course of the fifties the commission concluded that most of the problems encountered by medical inspectors in the field did not require medical training. Charges brought against a dispensary medical officer, for example, were rarely about malpractice. Usually they involved some aspect of dereliction of duty and could as well be adjudicated by a regular inspector as not.[25] On the other hand, regular inspectors were often asked to give an opinion on matters of public health which were more easily and effectively handled by a medical inspector. Moreover, when emergencies arose, such as the epidemics which struck certain localities in the western counties in the early 1860s, it was difficult to switch medical officers to them because of their involvement in normal duties. The commission therefore asked for the authority to empower regular poor law inspectors to take over the duties of the medical inspectors. Naturally this move triggered opposition in the medical community which interpreted it as the first step in a plan by the commission to phase out the medical inspectors altogether.[26] Well-prepared to defend their interests, the medical community ensured that the authorising legislation was delayed. The commission therefore extended to their medical inspectors the authority to function as regular inspectors, a move which gave them some of the flexibility they desired.[27] Full realisation of the intent of the commission was not achieved until 1868 when each class of inspector was authorised to act for the other, both being empowered to carry out

---

[24] PRO, Treasury papers, T. 165/1, x/j 8590. This document is part of a collection of briefs on the structure and function of various government departments, in this case the Irish Local Government Board, which were designed as an aid to ministers. The collection is commonly referred to as the 'Blue notes' and contains much useful information on the cost and development of government agencies in the Victorian era.

[25] Poor Law Commission to the lord lieutenant, 21 Feb. 1860, chief secretary's office, registered papers (CSO/RP) 1860/18567, This is a long letter explaining the commission's experience in dealing with medical officers who had been charged with dereliction of duty.

[26] DMP xxxix (1858), 235.

[27] Fifteenth and tenth annual report (HC 1862, xxiv), 562.

sanitary inspections under the provisions of the Sanitary Act of 1866.[28] From the commission's perspective these arrangements constituted a more efficient use of personnel. The medical men remained unconvinced.

The first task to which the medical inspectors had to apply themselves was the reorganisation of the dispensary system. On 12 November 1851 the Poor Law Commission issued an order instructing the boards of guardians to divide their unions into as many dispensary districts, according to area and population density, as the guardians thought appropriate. In many unions these districts could be created around existing facilities, although many of these dispensaries were found to be without funds, their subscribers having withdrawn due to the hardships imposed by the famine, and, consequently, the grand jury grants having lapsed as well. The commission, which supervised this process very closely, insisted on such institutions being shifted to the poor rate immediately.[29] In order to speed up the process some guardians authorised the commission to create districts for them. Those boards which formed their own were required to submit their proposals for the commission's approval. Occasionally it was denied, most often because the commissioners thought the proposed districts too large. Ever sensitive to the rates, guardians tended to prefer fewer rather than more districts in order to reduce the number of medical officers they would have to employ. In cases where the commissioners thought this tendency extreme they either insisted that the district in question be divided or that an additional medical officer be employed to share the duties.[30]

Under the Medical Charities Act each dispensary was subject to three overlapping but administratively distinct authorities: the Poor Law Commission, a board of guardians and a committee of management. Generally speaking the commission possessed the same kind of supervisory powers over dispensary relief that it exercised over ordinary pauper relief. Specifically this meant the commission defined the rules and regulations for the organisation and conduct of dispensary services, as provided by the statute, and systematically monitored the performance of each dispensary through its corps of inspectors and the scrutiny of the reports required of medical officers, committees of management and the guardians.[31] When clear violations or differences of opinion arose over matters of interpretation the commission had the final authority and could enforce compliance with its view by issuing an order under the seal of the lord lieutenant. The commission also had the power to determine the qualifications of medical officers and to approve their appointment and set their salaries.

On the local level supervision of the dispensaries was shared between

---

[28] *Twenty-second and seventeenth annual report* (HC 1868–9, xxviii), 378–9.

[29] First annual report of the commissioners for administering the laws for relief of the poor in Ireland under the Medical Charities Act (HC 1852–3, l), 335.

[30] Ibid. 336.

[31] 14 & 15 Vic., c. 68, *Statutes at large*, xci. 319.

boards of guardians and committees of management. The former were responsible for supervising the financial condition of each dispensary in their unions. Since there were 723 dispensary districts (in 1851) and 163 unions, most boards of guardians had between four and five districts to superintend.[32] They were required to furnish dispensary facilities either by constructing or renting an appropriate building, to furnish medicines and medical supplies, and to pay the medical officers and other dispensary personnel. The list of medicines and medical equipment was drawn up by the Irish Poor Law Commission. The guardians were expected to contract for these items with reputable suppliers. Medical officers were permitted to request special medicines and equipment not found on the master list. Provision of both medicines and equipment appears to have been generous by the standards of the time. John Lambert, an English poor law inspector who toured the Irish dispensaries in 1866, found the quantity and range of medical materials 'surprisingly large and varied'.[33] However, no food or spirits were to be given to dispensary patients. Anyone in need of these items was to apply at the local workhouse where he would be provided with sustenance through the normal channel of indoor relief.

The committees of management were the basic units of dispensary administration. Each district was governed by its own committee composed of local property owners. There were two classes of committee members: guardians who were resident in the district or who owned property there, and resident ratepayers who owned or occupied property valued at £30 per year or more. The guardians who fitted the above description were ex-officio members of the committee. Eligible ratepayers were appointed to each committee by the board of guardians. These appointments were always necessary because the Irish Poor Law Commission made it a point to encourage the participation of such men. If, as originally constituted, a given committee was composed of a disproportionately large number of ex-officio members, the commission, which had the authority to set the size of committees of management, simply required that the total be increased.[34]

The size of managing committees varied according to the area and population of the district. A typical example is provided by the Cork Union in 1851. It was a large union containing ten districts, nine of which were relatively small and rural and the other, Cork City, large and urban. The nine rural districts had committees ranging from nine to twenty-one members. The urban district had eight medical officers and a committee of sixty-six.[35] In 1861, ten years after the dispensary system was reorganised, the Irish Poor

---

[32] The maximum number of districts in a union was ten, of which there were two examples, and the minimum number was two, of which there were twenty-one examples: *First annual report*, 335–6.

[33] *Lambert report*, 581.

[34] *First annual report*, 337.

[35] Order declaring dispensary districts from the Poor Law Commission to the Board of

Law Commission reported that in the country as a whole managing committees were staffed by about 10,000 persons.[36]

The managing committees exercised control over dispensary medical relief in several ways. They supervised the operation of their dispensaries through fortnightly meetings at which they were supposed to review the dispensary records compiled since the previous meeting and hear the medical officer's report. Once a month they forwarded to the local board of guardians a report of their own on the numbers of cases treated and dispensary medicines and equipment consumed and on hand. Guardians subsequently submitted the collective statistics for the dispensary districts to the Poor Law Commission in Dublin. Managing committee members, as well as the poor law relieving officers and wardens, were also responsible for authorising medical treatment from the dispensary medical officer through the distribution of dispensary tickets to poor persons resident in the district who applied for them. Tickets were of two types, E-1 and E-2, commonly known as black and red tickets respectively, from the colour of their lettering.[37] A black ticket entitled the bearer to treatment and medicine at the dispensary itself. The red tickets were reserved for those persons too ill to appear at the dispensary and required the medical officer to call at the patients' homes.

Finally, the committees were empowered to appoint the medical officers. The qualifications for that post were of course defined by the Poor Law Commission which also reserved the right of final approval, but the local authorities were responsible for finding a medical officer who suited them. It could be a touchy business. One of the most frequent complaints about the grand jury system had been the lack of minimum standards of training and competence among the medical personnel. Under the Medical Charities Act the Poor Law Commission had been given the authority to define such standards. However, in 1852 the subject of professional qualifications for doctors and surgeons continued to be confusing as well as controversial and would not be simplified until the passage of the Medical Registration Act of 1858. Furthermore, some medical officers already in charge of existing dispensaries lacked widely recognised degrees or licences although they had served their communities faithfully and well for years. The decisions required of both the managing committees and the Poor Law Commission could therefore be very difficult. If the qualifications were interpreted too narrowly good men might well have been eliminated from positions for which their actual performance qualified them. On the other hand, the movement toward increased professionalism in medical circles was gaining momentum throughout the United Kingdom and could not be ignored. Article 5 of the commission's rules and regulations for the conduct of dispensaries stipulated

Guardians, Cork Union, No. 16,739/52, Cork Archives Council, Cork union order and circular book, 1852.

[36] *Fourteenth and ninth annual report* (HC 1861, xxvii), appendix A, 384.

[37] *First annual report*, 338.

the requirements for medical officers and reflected these contemporary complexities.

Dispensary medical officers were to be at least twenty-three years old and qualified to practise in surgery, medicine and midwifery. As in the past the emphasis was upon surgical skills. A candidate was to have the licence of the Irish Royal College of Surgeons or the degree of some other 'College or Body' in Great Britain or Ireland.[38] No similar licence or diploma from any of the Irish or British colleges of physicians was specifically required, it only being necessary that the candidate be 'licensed to practice as a "Medical Man" '. Broad as these requirements were some existing medical officers could not meet them. The commission therefore added the provision that it reserved the right to exempt anyone it deemed fit from the above requirements on the basis of its own judgement.[39]

Through the application of this provision most of the medical officers who had been employed in the dispensaries before the passage of the Medical Charities Act were retained in their positions.[40] The question of qualifications for dispensary MOs was eventually simplified by the Medical Registration Act of 1858 which provided that after 1 January 1859 'no person shall hold any appointment as a physician, surgeon or other medical officer either in the military or navy or in emigrant vessels or any hospital, infirmary, dispensary, or lying in hospital not supported wholly by voluntary contributions or in any asylum, workhouse, etc., unless he be registered under this act'.[41]

Medical officers employed under the Poor Law Commission were given six months from the passage of the act to register. Degrees and licences from all the major Irish, Scottish and English schools constituted appropriate credentials for registration and the process could be completed by mail. A registration office was established at the College of Surgeons in Dublin and was administered by Henry Maunsell. By this time all dispensary medical officers with questionable credentials had apparently either resigned or retired because there is no record of anyone failing to qualify under the new regime.

However, the 1858 act did eventually produce a major change in the requirements for dispensary medical officers. In January 1860 the Irish College of Physicians brought to the attention of the Poor Law Commission the fact that the English Poor Law Board had altered its regulations and now required medical officers to possess a degree in medicine as well as surgery. The Irish College argued that this was in accordance with Clause 31 of the Medical Act which stated that 'every person registered under this act shall be

---

[38] Form of order declaring dispensary districts, art. 5, 'Qualifications of medical officers', ibid. appendix A, no. 7, 354.
[39] Ibid.
[40] *Royal Commission report*, appendix ii, 301.
[41] Registration under the Medical Act, *Seventh annual report* (HC 1859, session 1, ix), appendix A, no. 11, 364.

entitled according to his qualifications to practice medicine or surgery or medicine and surgery, as the case may be, in any part of Her Majesty's dominions'.[42] They went on to note that both the army and navy medical departments now required both degrees and that the East India Company required an examination in medicine. The Irish College therefore requested that the Poor Law Commission make a similar alteration in the requirements for its workhouse and dispensary MOs.

Naturally, the Irish College of Surgeons, which had always considered its licenciates qualified in medicine as well as surgery, made strenuous efforts to retain its dominion over poor law medical positions. But the Poor Law Commission had been convinced by the weight of the physicians' arguments that proper medical degrees were important for its medical officers, especially those practising alone in distant provincial posts. Consequently, beginning in 1863, both licences were necessary for medical officers working alone. If two or more officers worked in together it was only necessary that between them they hold both credentials.

Generally speaking the basic duties of MOs were unchanged under the Medical Charities Act. They were to be present at the dispensary on the days and at such hours as the committee of management directed and to treat all persons who appeared there and presented proper tickets.[43] Furthermore, they were to call promptly at the homes and provide treatment for those persons who submitted visiting tickets. For most medical officers these duties constituted the bulk of their obligations. However, there were innovations under the new act. For one thing the vaccination arrangements were changed. The old contract system was abandoned and in its place a more comprehensive system was adopted. Each officer was required to vaccinate free of charge every person who requested it. No tickets were necessary. Vaccine was to be paid for by the guardians but the MOs received no remuneration for successful vaccinations as they had under the previous system.

Dispensary MOs were also to examine and certify any 'dangerous lunatic' brought before a justice of the peace within the district if the justice so ordered. Moreover, if a bridewell or house of correction under the control of the Poor Law Commission were located in the district, the MO was required to treat and supply medicine to the inmates. Again, as in the case of vaccination, no special or extra payment was forthcoming for the performance of these duties. However, if in the opinion of the Poor Law Commission, such extraordinary services were exceptionally demanding, they should be taken into consideration when fixing the salaries of MOs in such districts.

Perhaps the most conspicuous and comprehensive change in the routine

---

[42] Correspondence on the qualifications of medical officers, no. 1, Letter for the King and Queens College of Physicians to the Poor Law Commission, 30 Jan. 1860, *Sixteenth and eleventh annual report* (HC 1863, xxii), appendix C, III, 552.

[43] Orders, circulars, instructions, no. 28, General rules for the government of dispensary districts, *First annual report*, appendix A, 378.

of the MOs instituted under the new system involved the keeping of records. No records at all had actually been required under the grand jury system. In fact many dispensaries had kept some statistics on cases treated and monies expended for the benefit of subscribers, but no uniform, detailed and nation-wide statistics on dispensary relief had been compiled. The Poor Law Commission was determined to remedy this situation. True to its utilitarian view that precise and comprehensive medical statistics were essential in order to gain a true picture of the nation's health and to detect epidemics in time to take effective preventive action, it directed each MO to keep a thorough set of records, including a medical relief register, a vaccination register, a case book and a report book as well as alphabetical indices to the registers and the case book. M'Donnell, the medical commissioner, estimated it would take half-an-hour per day to maintain these records.[44] The books were subject to regular examination and the MOs were also required to make monthly reports to the committee of management detailing cases treated, medicines consumed, additional duties performed, etc. The drudgery of this work came to constitute one of the principal and continuing grievances of the medical officers. Although the commission gradually lightened the load, it remained adamant that it be done.

Aside from the medical officers some of the larger dispensaries also employed additional personnel such as compounders and/or midwives. The former had to be qualifed as apothecaries or pharmaceutical chemists, or to have served as compounders in the army medical service for at least four years. Their major duties were to prepare prescriptions and maintain the drug cabinet. The midwives had to be at least twenty-three years old and to have a certificate from a recognised lying-in hospital. They assisted the MOs in their obstetrical duties or delivered babies themselves.

The reorganisation of the dispensary system was completed with the approval of the Tralee Union plan on 27 May 1852. In the months following the passage of the Medical Charities Act the *Dublin Medical Press* had frequently expressed the fear that the new system would be more limited than the old one, an anxiety based on Somerville's promise of economy.[45] As it turned out it was substantially larger. A total of 723 districts had been created comprising 960 separate dispensaries served by 776 medical officers and ten midwives. The fact that dispensaries outnumbered districts was due to the need for more than one building in the larger districts where the distances from outlying regions to the main dispensary would have proved a real hardship for some of the residents. At its peak the grand jury system had never consisted of more than 668 dispensaries and had not existed at all in some parts of the country. The Poor Law Commission was pleased with the new arrangements. In concluding its first report it observed that

---

[44] J. M. M'Donnell to Lord Naas, 5 June 1852, Mayo Papers, MS 11020,
[45] *DMP* xxvi (1851), 126.

by the proceedings taken under the Medical Charities Act, a system of Extern Medical Relief heretofore imperfectly developed in Ireland, resting on a financial basis at once uncertain in regard to its continuance and partial in its pressure as a tax and unattended with any definite responsibilities on the part of the agents principally concerned in its administration has been exchanged for a system uniform in its arrangements and universal in the scope of its operation, supported everywhere, according to the exigency of the case, by funds levied under the laws existing for the Relief of the Destitute Poor, and vitally influenced in its administration by well defined and practical responsibilities under the direction and control of a central authority.[46]

In the course of the next two decades the dispensary system was expanded in both facilities and services. Relying on encouragement and recommendation to the guardians for the most part, but prepared to be firm if necessary, the commission insisted on the steady upgrading of medical services. As problems or inequities were brought to its attention by the medical inspectors, the commission obtained increases in facilities and personnel. Ordinarily the local committees and boards of guardians were co-operative. Recommendations by the commission that districts be divided or combined in order to provide more effective medical care in areas found in practice to be poorly served were often readily accepted by the union authorities. The same was true of the appointment of additional medical officers or midwives. Occasionally the guardians balked at such demands in which case the commission was frequently prepared to insist on increases by issuing an order under seal. One especially defiant board of guardians had to be taken before the Queen's Bench before the commission got its way.[47] That it would go to such lengths is indicative not only of the authority of the Poor Law Commission but also of its dedication to its medical role.

By 1872 the effect of the changes was apparent. While dispensary districts had been consolidated slightly from 723 to 719, a reflection of the loss of population over the preceeding twenty years, 111 dispensaries had been added, bringing the total to 1,071. In terms of personnel the number of apothecaries had remained the same (38), but 78 medical officers and 177 midwives had been added to bring the totals to 801 and 187 respectively. Moreover, expenditures for dispensary services had expanded even more rapidly than personnel. In 1852–3, the first full year of operation, the dispensary system cost £88,440. In its annual report for that year the Poor Law Commission assured the government that expenditures under the Medical Charities Act would not exceed £100,000 in any given year.[48] Nevertheless, the tendency for the commission to support the improvement of their medical services proved to be stronger than their well-known predilection for

---

46 *First annual report*, 348.
47 See the case of the guardians of Ballinasloe Union: *Seventh annual report*, 342–3.
48 *First annual report*, 346.

economy. Though couched in apologetic tones, the annual reports chronicle the steady addition of dispensaries here and medical officers there with the concurrent necessity for ever larger budgets. Even leaving aside for the moment the additional costs of the expanded vaccination programme, which was included in the medical charities budgets, dispensary costs rose to £127,362 by 1871–2.[49]

Moreover, these increases become more impressive when it is borne in mind that the Irish population was falling steadily in these years. Although the 1850s and 1860s were decades of economic growth and prosperity in Ireland, especially when compared with the first half of the century, the effect of the famine on landholding patterns was toward fewer but larger units. Thus, even though the population had been drastically reduced by the famine, the continued consolidation of holdings meant fewer and fewer Irishmen could realistically hope for farms and families of their own. Emigration increased and marriage rates declined. The 6.6 million of 1851 dropped to 5.4 million by 1871, a trend continuing well into the twentieth century.[50]

Reduced population meant that the ratio of dispensary facilities and personnel to potential patients increased more rapidly than the raw data on the growth of the system alone would suggest. For example, in 1852–3 there was one medical officer for every 8,400 persons and one dispensary for every 6,820. Twenty years later the proportions had shifted to one for every 6,800 persons and one dispensary for every 5,300. Or to look at it yet another way, while the population was declining by 18 per cent between 1851 and 1871, expenditure on dispensary relief was increasing by 44 per cent. These figures testify to the improvement in availability of both dispensaries and medical personnel. Equally important to an understanding of the extended reach of the dispensary system in these years is an appreciation of the fact that it was, as in the grand jury days, non-pauperising.

Matters were significantly different in England where poor law medical relief was confined to that same class of people that qualified for all other forms of relief – the unpropertied and chronically unemployed paupers at the bottom of the social ladder. The merely poor did not qualify for poor law medical care. They were not without resources since England had many private charitable hospitals, infirmaries and dispensaries. Yet they had no right to state medical relief. In Ireland this dichotomy did not exist, or at least did not exist in anything like the same form. A few voluntary dispensaries, mainly in Dublin, survived the Medical Charities Act and the county infirmaries had stayed independant of poor law control. But in general medi-

---

[49] *Annual report of the Local Government Board for Ireland being the first report under 'The Local Government Board (Ireland) Act'* (HC 1873, xxix), 443. Statistics of this sort appear in all the annual reports. Hereafter, with the exception of special compilations of figures which appear from time to time, the reader is to assume the figures are from the report for the year following the date of their occurrence.

[50] B. R. Mitchell and Phyllis Deane, *Abstract of British historical statistics*, London 1962, 9.

cal charity in Ireland had been state subsidised from its inception and, consequently, there had been one rather than two classes of medical charity in Ireland. Under such conditions division of the poor into paupers and the rest made no sense. The early medical charities reformers saw this non-pauperising principle as a strength of the system and urged its retention.[51] Consequently, when transferral of the medical charities to the Poor Law Commission became a serious possibility, the commission found it had to accommodate itself to this condition. Evidence of the commission's willingness to accept non-pauperising medical care was provided as early as 1841. George Nicholls's report of that year, based on the survey conducted by Denis Phelan, observed that while it was clear parliament intended free medical relief for the sick poor in Ireland to be confined to those persons absolutely without capacity to pay, it 'may be impossible always to discriminate between this class and the one immediately above it and in a condition to contribute moderately; and under existing circumstances it is perhaps right that the latter class should also be supplied with gratuitous Medical Relief'.[52] The medical charities bill based on Nicholls's report and introduced by Lord Eliot in the following year incorporated this view as did all its successors.

The Medical Charities Act of 1851 did not mention the word 'destitute', substituting instead the ambiguous expression 'poor persons', a category which could easily encompass a substantial segment of Irish society. Moreover, the act did not furnish any specific criteria by which to determine who was to be considered a poor person, nor did the Poor Law Commission offer any guidelines for making such judgements in its dispensary rules and regulations. Interpretation was left solely to the dispensary committee men responsible for allocating dispensary tickets. In each individual case the issuer of the ticket was required to use his discretion regarding the qualifications of the applicant who stood before him. In the absence of guidance from the statute and bearing in mind the fact that local rates paid for the medical care and that local committee men presumably knew best who among their community were deserving and who were not, the commission left the burden of decision on the local level.[53] The only check against excessive or corrupt distribution of tickets was an appeal to the committee. If, in their collective judgement, a recipient was clearly unqualified to receive dispensary relief, they had the authority to cancel the ticket and require payment for any services rendered.

In practice the definition of poor persons was liberally interpreted. In the first year of operation the dispensaries treated over 690,000 persons, or approximately 11 per cent of the population. In the course of the 1850s and early 1860s the number of dispensary cases increased steadily to a peak of

---

[51] See above ch. ii.
[52] *Poor Law Commission report* (1841), 13.
[53] *Royal Commission report*, appendix ii, 298–9.

almost 890,000 cases in 1863–4, nearly 16 per cent of the population. The high totals of the early sixties corresponded with successive failures of the potato crop in the western counties.[54] Although not as severe as the failures which produced the great famine, they did generate a period of hard times. Subsequently dispensary cases declined gradually to 720,000 in 1871–2. Given the sustained emigration of the Irish, that still amounted to more than 13 per cent of the population.

Comparison of these totals with those compiled under the grand juries is difficult because of the weakness of the records kept during that period. The figure most often given for persons treated in the whole medical charities system in any given year during the thirties and forties is around a million. The bulk of these were dispensary patients, one supposes, though fever hospital and infirmary statistics were included as well. A more significant problem concerning comparability lies in the fact that contemporary investigators considered the figures too high owing to the tendency for medical officers to count prescriptions rather than patients.[55] Since one patient could be given several prescriptions dispensary statistics were inflated, a useful way of impressing subscribers and grand jurors perhaps. Under the Medical Charities Act statistics for dispensary relief were based upon the number of tickets issued. Since one ticket was supposed to guarantee treatment until the patient was either cured or died, regardless of how many prescriptions it may have taken, the correspondence between individual patients and tickets was probably fairly even.[56] It is probable, therefore, that the reformed dispensaries treated as many patients as their predecessors, and they may have treated more. Given the decline in population, the percentage of the total population which used them was undoubtedly very much greater.

Who were the 'poor persons'? Who really used the dispensaries? Breaking down the figures for dispensary use in terms of social classes is also fraught with difficulties. No records were kept of the financial or social condition of dispensary patients either before or after the Medical Charities Act. None the less a great deal of more or less informed opinion exists on the subject. Clearly both agricultural and unskilled workers and their families fitted the criteria for poor persons and these groups must have made up the bulk of the patients treated. However, the ambiguity of the qualifications meant that many persons who were somewhat better off frequently resorted to the dis-

---

[54] See particularly the *Fourteenth and ninth annual report*, 318.

[55] *Poor Law Commission report* (1841), 2.

[56] The Irish Poor Law Commission made a point of insisting that a single dispensary ticket entitled its bearer to all the treatment necessary to obtain complete recovery from the ailment, if possible. Dispensary committees and medical officers were informed that 'A dispensary ticket continues in force until it is cancelled by the committee, or as long as the patient continues to present himself at the dispensary in the case of an E-1 ticket, or until the patient recovers or terminates in the case of visiting or E-2 tickets': *First annual report*, 398.

pensary system as well. One particularly well-informed authority observed that even most artisans, domestic and indoor servants, small farmers and petty tradesmen could receive gratuitous medical care because their circumstances could vary so much from year to year.[57] The receipt of free medicines and treatment by such persons generated controversy and opposition.

By the late 1860s the extent of outdoor medical care afforded by the dispensaries had assumed alarming proportions in the view of some observers. John Lambert, the English Poor Law inspector who visited Ireland in 1866 specifically to evaluate the dispensary system, went so far as to describe the distribution of tickets as 'lavish' and cautioned the English Poor Law Board against such practices in the event of the dispensary system being adopted there.[58] Complaints against presumed exploitation of the system emanated from Ireland too. A particularly interesting and imaginative criticism appeared in 1867 when the parliamentary reform bill was under consideration. It not only sheds some light on the question of what kinds of people used the dispensaries but suggests the lengths to which opponents would go to curtail such use. Lord Naas, then chief secretary for the Conservative administration, received a copy of a letter sent to Disraeli by a certain Charles N. Davis, a member of a Belfast dispensary committee and an ardent Tory.[59] Davis professed to be appalled at the scale of dispensary relief. He stated that within the last four months up to 35,000 prescriptions and around 7,000 house calls had been provided by dispensary medical officers in the Belfast dispensary districts alone. He estimated that 3–4,000 rated occupiers of small tenements regularly received treatment under the Medical Charities Act. Given the democratic tendencies of the new reform bill he proposed that a clause be inserted disenfranchising dispensary users. Such a measure, he assured Disraeli, would save some of the Irish boroughs for the Conservative cause for, he went on, 'from my own knowledge of the Cities of Dublin, Cork, Waterford, Wexford and other Boroughs in Ireland it would be the means of disenfranchising thousands, for the poorer classes never think of paying either for Medicine or Medical attendance as long as those dispensaries are in existence'.[60] The Davis letter was brought to Naas's attention by a Dublin acquaintance, Mr John Norwood, who himself urged the chief secretary to take it seriously, noting that in his opinion the abuses of the Medical Charities Act were not exaggerated. Norwood concluded that if Naas acted, 'your

---

[57] *Royal Commission report*, appendix ii, 298.

[58] *Lambert report*, 582.

[59] Richard Southwell Bourke (1822–72), sixth earl of Mayo, was known for most of his career by the courtesy title of Lord Naas. A prominent Irish Conservative, Naas was chief secretary on three separate occasions, 1852–3, 1858–9 and 1866–7. He was a moderate Tory who favoured state support for education and public health. He was sponsor of the Irish Vaccination Act of 1858: *DNB* ii. 919–22.

[60] Copy of a letter from Charles N. Davis to Benjamin Disraeli, 15 Mar. 1867, Mayo papers, MS 11157.

Lordship would have the aid and good wishes of the medical profession throughout the country and save much cost to the ratepayers'.[61]

Norwood was quite right about the attitude of the Irish doctors. It is worth considering for a moment why they found the administration of the dispensaries by the Poor Law Commission unsatisfactory. The ease with which tickets were acquired was one criticism, of course, but they were also put out by the judicial power of the commission and by the low levels of their own salaries.

The matter of their remuneration was never adequately arranged in the view of the medical officers. In the mid-fifties salaries averaged less than £80 annually. Some were over £100 but many were much less. The salaries, set by the commission itself, were calculated on the basis of the size of the dispensary district, both in terms of area and population, and the prospects the medical officer might have for private practice. The doctors felt £100 ought to have been set as a minimum annual amount and that it ought to be higher still in those poor, remote, sparsely populated yet gigantic districts characteristic of the western and southern counties, where dispensary service constituted the bulk of the medical officer's work and income.[62] This grievance was never dealt with to the doctors' satisfaction although the average wage did increase to the £100 level by the end of the 1860s.

A large portion of the rise was a product of legislation which came into operation in 1867 and defrayed half of the medical officer's wages out of the consolidated fund, an arrangement enjoyed by the English poor law medical officers for many years previously.[63] The *Dublin Medical Press* had been calling for a grant of this type since 1853.[64] Once it had been approved Power made a considerable effort to have the lion's share of the grant allocated to the poorest districts instead of being distributed evenly.[65] But uniform distribution was the practice in England and the Treasury insisted on the same arrangement in Ireland.[66] In spite of these increases Irish medical officers considered themselves ill-used well into the twentieth century.[67]

---

[61] Norwood to Naas, May 14 1867, ibid.

[62] *DMP* 1852–66, passim. Until the *DMP* combined with the *Medical Circular* in 1866 and moved its headquarters to London, it remained a strong supporter of the Irish poor law medical officers and virtually every issue contains some article or letter bearing upon their complaints, especially regarding salaries.

[63] PRO, Treasury papers, T. 165/1, x/j 8590, 7. The average sum each dispensary medical officer received under the 1866–7 grant amounted to £44. 'One of the main objects of the grant', the Treasury brief observes, 'is to induce local authorities to be more liberal in their administration of medical relief to the poor'.

[64] *DMP* xxx (1853), 27.

[65] Correspondence on medical and educational grant, *Twenty-first and sixteenth annual report* (HC 1867–8, xxxiii), appendix A, II, 457–9.

[66] Ibid.

[67] *Royal Commission report*, appendix ii, 301–10. By 1906 the average salary for a dispensary medical officer had increased to £116 per year plus vaccination and birth registration fees, but it was still regarded as inadequate and unprogressive.

The legal authority held by the Poor Law Commission over its employees was another matter which the medical personnel resented. Under the Medical Charities Act the commission was empowered to conduct its own investigations into charges brought against any of its medical officers and, if convinced of the validity of the charges, could summarily dismiss that officer with the added proviso that he was never to hold office under the commission again. Such investigations and judgements took place *in camera* and were beyond appeal. These powers were used on a number of occasions in the 1850s producing growing resentment among the officers who came to feel Star Chamber methods were being employed. They demanded that hearings be opened to the public, that trial by jury replace trial by tribunal, and that simple dismissal be made the most severe penalty.[68] But as late as 1872 no modification of the rules had been made.

Finally, the medical officers became increasingly disturbed by what they came to consider rampant abuse of dispensary ticket distribution by committee men. Two aspects of the problem particularly concerned them: (1) excessive distribution of red tickets, which required the medical officer to visit the patient, often in a remote corner of the district; and (2) the use of dispensary services by persons, who in the opinion of the medical officers, were perfectly able to afford treatment and medicines. There were grotesque examples of the latter. As in the old days retail tradesmen who happened to be committee men were known to have signed entire books of tickets and left them with their clerks to distribute among the customers in order to encourage business.[69] One committee man was petty enough to have obtained three months' supply of cod liver oil from the dispensary by the ruse of sending his child to get it under an assumed name. Then there were the landlords who gave out tickets to their servants. Medical officers felt that persons of such affluence should pay for medical attention for their retainers, though the use of dispensary committee status in this way was often considered an ancient and time-honoured prerogative.

While the above examples represented corruption of the worst kind the medical officers recognised that many cases of ticket abuse derived from carelessness rather than premeditation. Too many committeemen, in the opinion of the medical officers, failed to investigate the circumstances of persons whom they did not know well who appealed to them for tickets.[70] When faced with the bearer of such a ticket officers were required under the statute to honour it regardless of their suspicions. Only later could they appeal to the committee for cancellation. The trouble with that procedure, in their view, was that it worked less and less satisfactorily as time went on.

---

[68] *Freeman's Journal*, 29 Oct. 1859 (clipping in the Larcom papers, MS 7780).

[69] *Lambert report*, 582.

[70] See the report on the annual meeting of the Irish Medical Association, *DMP* xl (1858), 372.

In the early 1850s cancellations had been comparatively high, over 12,000 in the three years 1852–4.[71] Thereafter, they fell off steadily year by year. In 1865 only 828 cancellations were recorded and by 1872 the total was down to 488. Given that there were never fewer than 720,000 tickets distributed in those years, the medical officers appear to have had a point. Several factors account for this development, one being the responsibility of the Irish medical profession itself.

Throughout the nineteenth century Irish physicians and surgeons continued to insist upon the traditional guinea fee from private patients.[72] Some doctors, of course, reduced or waived that charge as an act of individual charity, but the tradition was very strong and was apparently tied to the profession's sense of dignity. The probability that the guinea would be required forced many persons to seek medical treatment in the dispensaries even if they would have preferred to go elsewhere. The question any dispensary committee had to ask in considering the cancellation of a ticket was therefore whether or not the recipient could afford the guinea. In 1868 it was estimated that the average wage in Ireland amounted to about 7s. per week, a substantial improvement over earlier wage levels and indicative of a new prosperity in the country.[73] But this means that even under improved economic conditions the guinea charge amounted to fully three weeks wages, an impossible amount for the working class and even the lower middle class, one suspects.

However, the failure of the cancellation provisions was not simply the result of the doctors' excessive fee structure. A basic feature of the dispensary service, which tended to work against the medical personnel, was the fact that they were paid fixed salaries rather than per patient fees. The inherent dynamics of such a system led the committee men to increase the use of the poor law doctors. As long as the Irish medical profession produced such an abundance of practitioners that dispensary positions were seen as desirable, in spite of their many and obvious disadvantages, and disgruntled MOs easily replaced, then the ticket distributors were in a commanding position. The interest of both ratepayers and the Poor Law Commission was served by extracting as much labour from the MOs as possible at a minimum cost. From time to time some sort of fee system for visiting (red) tickets was proposed, but the commission professed to prefer the simplicities of fixed salaries.[74]

---

[71] Cancellation figures are provided in the statistical appendices at the end of each annual report. They were never accumulated historically and each report must therefore be consulted separately.

[72] *Royal Commission report*, appendix ii, 299. See also *Lambert report*, 582. The practice remained a problem for the poor on into the twentieth century.

[73] *Twenty-first and sixteenth annual report*, 426.

[74] For example, in 1859 the Irish Poor Law Commission received requests from two boards of guardians that legislation be passed enabling dispensary committees to fix fees to be paid on tickets issued to small landholders. The commission replied that such a scale

Furthermore, it seems probable that the very high cancellation figures in the early fifties were at least in part due to the inexperience of dispensary committee men, many of whom had never participated in medical charity in the past. On the other hand, it must be borne in mind that during and immediately following the famine the poor rates were very high and local authorities especially anxious to reduce costs. However, as the decade unfolded Ireland began to experience unprecedented prosperity, the up side of the famine catastrophe whereby, once out of the ruck of misery and disease, the land and its industry had far fewer people to support. By 1860 the poor rates had fallen dramatically and it is evident that the guardians felt able to relax the restrictions formerly exercised in the allocation of poor relief in general and dispensary relief in particular. Certainly the statistics show a marked increase in outdoor relief in the late sixties clearly indicative of a greater generosity than had prevailed earlier. This factor undoubtedly played a role in the growing reluctance to cancel dispensary tickets as well. The ratio of indoor to outdoor relief in Ireland was a subject which generated a good deal of controversy in the late fifties and one which shed light on the metamorphosis of the Poor Law Commission into a medical care rather than a strictly poor relief agency.

In the two decades following the great famine the commission placed greater emphasis upon indoor relief than either of its parallel institutions in Scotland and England. Alfred Power, true to his early education in such doctrine at the hands of Edwin Chadwick, was convinced of its value. In his view it combined the dual advantages of completely satisfying the material needs of the recipient while simultaneously permitting the poor law authority to maximise its control of expenditure.[75] Outdoor relief he felt to be insufficient and largely uncontrollable. Under the extraordinary conditions imposed by the famine massive outdoor relief had been unavoidable at the time Power had taken control of the commission in 1849. But as the crops improved in the following years he encouraged the resumption of a regimen of virtually total indoor relief. In 1849 fully 1,210,482 persons had been on the outdoor relief rolls. Ten years later a mere 5,425 persons received such assistance while 183,706 were provided for in the workhouses.[76]

Power was proud of this achievment, especially as it attracted attention in other sections of the United Kingdom. The annual report of the Scottish poor law administration for 1859 contained a comparison of the Scottish and Irish systems much to the credit of the latter. In a note to Larcom, Power recommended the report and reflected that the Scottish system had been adopted on the recommendation of a royal commission of which Twistleton

would 'unsettle' the present system of remunerating medical officers by salary: Poor Law Commission to Lord Naas, 9 Apr. 1859, Mayo papers, MS 11030,

[75] For a full exposition of Power's views see his short pamphlet *A paper on outdoor relief in Ireland: prepared at Earl Spencer's request*, London 1875.

[76] *Fourteenth and ninth annual report* (HC 1861, xxviii), appendix A, IV, 382.

had been a dissenting member. Twistleton, Power's predecessor as head of the Poor Law Commission, had recommended the Irish system but his views had been rejected. Power concluded 'they are now beginning to feel their mistake after a trial of thirteen years during which expenditure has gradually risen to £640,000 with a certainty of further increases'.[77]

Not all close observers of Irish poor relief drew the same sanguine conclusions as Power. In 1859 Denis Phelan, now retired but alert and plucky as ever, published a pamphlet attacking the heavy insistence on indoor relief. Phelan was distressed by differences between poor law policy in England and Scotland and that in Ireland. Using statistics drawn from recent annual reports of these agencies he showed that in the former two countries outdoor relief now constituted the overwhelming bulk of all poor law aid. In 1857 the average daily number of persons receiving such care amounted to 705,587 in England and 113,434 in Scotland while in Ireland the figure was but 954.[78] Put another way, of the entire English population 3.95 per cent were on outdoor relief and in Scotland the percentage was 3.7. By comparison the percentage of Irish getting outdoor relief was absurdly small, amounting to only 0.016 per cent. Expenditure reflected the same contrast. The poor law cost English ratepayers more than 6s. apiece, the Scottish ratepayers more than 4s., and their Irish counterparts only 1s. 7d. Phelan and other critics demanded greater outdoor relief in Ireland as well.

Such comparisons were useful as weapons with which to attack the Poor Law Commission but in several respects they gave a misleading impression of the real costs of Irish poor relief. First, they ignored the dispensary system which was not counted by either the commission or its critics as outdoor relief though in the broadest sense it certainly was. Critics left it out because not to have included it would have weakened their argument. In 1857 nearly 13 per cent of the Irish population had used the dispensaries. But the critics could be forgiven their oversight since the commission did not invoke dispensary care in its defence either. The commission considered its actions under the Medical Charities Act as completely separate from its other poor law obligations and never included them, even in the most general sense, as related to outdoor relief. Until 1860 completely separate reports were prepared for conventional poor relief and medical charities relief and, even after the reports were combined in that year, they were always confined to separate sections.

To the Poor Law Commission 'poor relief' meant total relief – food, clothing, fuel, shelter – all the essentials for life. It could be provided either in the workhouse, in which case these things were provided directly, or outdoors via some kind of monetary supplement to the recipient. Poor relief of this kind

[77] Power to Larcom, 23 March 1859, Larcom Papers, MS 7783.
[78] Denis Phelan, *Reform of the poor law system in Ireland or facts and observations on the inadequacies of the existing system of poor relief*, Dublin 1859, 2.

was confined strictly to paupers while medical relief was extended to poor persons. In the thinking of the commission the distinction was crucial. Any confusion of the two would produce the situation found in England where the poor rates were skyrocketing and control over the use of relief funds was much less secure. The annual reports underlined the fact that while total poor law expenditures were much lower in Ireland, expenditure per recipient was much higher.[79]

But the whole argument over indoor versus outdoor relief was misleading in another respect as well. Careful scrutiny of the figures demonstrated that in Ireland even indoor relief was ceasing to be applied largely to the able-bodied poor as was originally intended. Instead it was increasingly coming to be a form of medical relief too. This was partly because the workhouses were rapidly becoming homes for the aged and chronically ill. In 1851 statistics on admissions show that 34.8 per cent of workhouse inmates were able-bodied men and women and another 44.4 per cent were children under fifteen, while only 6.8 per cent were listed as aged and infirm.[80] However, the pattern altered in the following two decades. By 1871 the first two categories had declined to 15.9 per cent and 26.6 per cent respectively while the figure for the aged and infirm had climbed to 24.3 per cent. But even more important for our purposes, the workhouse infirmaries were being transformed into general hospitals treating both accident cases and non-contagious diseases. In 1851 only 14 per cent of workhouse inmates were admitted in sickness while by 1871 the figure had ballooned to fully 33.2 per cent.[81] The drift toward increasing the medical functions of the workhouses in part reflected a significant decrease in able-bodied pauperism, but it was also due to a premeditated effort on the part of the Poor Law Commission to expand the scope of its hospital services.

From the very beginnings of the agitation over the medical charities in the mid-1830s reformers had pressed for the creation of a comprehensive medical relief system. The Poor Inquiry Commission report, Phelan's pamphlet and subsequent poor law and parliamentary committee reports called for the establishment of a network of facilities which would incorporate the existing county infirmaries, district fever hospitals and the dispensaries.[82] Every medical charities bill up to and including the original version of the 1851 measure had been conceived along these lines. However, as we have seen, the oppo-

---

[79] The average annual expenditure on each pauper relieved in Ireland amounted to almost £10. In England the figure was less than £7 while in Scotland it was around £5. Neither expenditures nor persons relieved under the Medical Charities Act were included in these calculations: *Fourteenth and ninth annual report*, appendix A, IV, 386.

[80] *Twenty-fourth and nineteenth annual report* (HC 1871, xxviii), 2.

[81] Ibid. On the general process of the transformation of the workhouses into hospitals I have found Patricia Kelly, 'From workhouse to hospital: the role of the Irish workhouse in medical relief to 1922', unpubl. MA diss. London 1972, most useful.

[82] See chapter 2.

sition of the infirmary surgeons had forced Somerville to drop all but the dispensaries from the final version of that bill in order to get it through parliament. None the less, he and his associates in the Poor Law Commission were convinced of the desirability of eventually gaining control of the rest of the medical charities and fully intended to do so at the first opportunity.[83] It therefore came as no surprise to anyone familiar with these matters when in its annual report issued in the spring of 1854 the commission expressed its intention to submit a bill to parliament calling for the absorption of the county infirmaries and fever hospitals then still under the grand juries.

At this time the provincial hospitals in Ireland consisted of thirty-two county infirmaries, two infirmaries in Cork, one in Limerick and the so-called leper hospital in Waterford which, despite its name, had in fact been a general hospital for most of the century. The poor law authority conceded that these institutions had excellent personnel and provided good service but, reiterating the charges made on countless occasions in the past, argued that they lacked uniformity of management and control and were badly distributed about the country. Consequently, many people derived no benefit from them even though taxed for their upkeep.[84]

The grand jury fever hospitals were open to the same objections. The Poor Law Commission calculated that 84 per cent of their patients came from within a five-mile radius of each institution. In any case, as we have seen, the financial strain of the famine years had destroyed the bulk of these places. By 1854 only thirty-seven were left while the commission itself administered 146. The case for consolidation was therefore very strong.

The commission recommended that the poor law unions, of which there were 163 at the time, be made the unit for administration and taxation for both general and fever hospitals. The average area of each of the unions was equivalent to a circle with an eight-mile radius. Though not as desirable as the five-mile radius the new arrangements would be a considerable improvement on existing conditions. The commission argued that these arrangements were almost completed for the fever hospitals already and that the system was almost universal in operation. Buildings constructed during the famine would be adequate to serve as general hospitals and could be partially staffed by medical personnel already employed by the unions in dispensary and workhouse infirmary positions. Furthermore, as with the dispensaries, poor persons rather than paupers were to be admitted, a fundamental break with traditional workhouse practice. The addition of such hospital services, the commission felt, would provide Ireland with a medical care system which 'in point of organisation may be more comprehensive than any in Europe at present'.[85]

---

[83] Somerville to Clarendon, 27 July 1851, Clarendon Papers, Box 28.
[84] *Second annual report* (HC 1854, xx), 226–9.
[85] Ibid. 229.

But, as with medical charities bills of the past, proposing a measure and passing it were two different matters. It was to be eight years before the Poor Law Commission was legally permitted to run a hospital system of its own, and even then it would not include the country infirmaries or grand jury fever hospitals. By 1854 it had been three years since the dispensaries had been shifted to the Poor Law Commission. The desperate financial conditions which had made the change seem not only necessary but attractive had now long since passed, replaced by an increasingly vocal resentment of the nature of poor law administration. The medical officers chafed under what they considered to be excessive demands upon their time and energy – too much record keeping, too many red tickets, districts too large to move about in easily, and, worst of all, too little remuneration. The infirmary surgeons, historically hostile to any threat to the *status quo*, were once again in the vanguard of resistance to the latest Poor Law Commission threat. The *Dublin Medical Press*, which had been uncharacteristically moderate in its treatment of the operation of the Medical Charities Act since 1851, reverted to form in an editorial of 17 May 1854:

> It is now twenty years since the first campaign against the Irish Medical Charities was opened by the poor-law pioneers with appendix B, a formidable blue folio, . . . and from that time to the present hour, has the war against our institutions raged with implacable hostility. . . . [cooperation and forbearance have resulted only in] . . . fresh aggressions. . . . [recalling the struggles of 1837 and 1843]. . . . Let no man tell us that it is useless to contend with an inevitable destiny, or to resist an overwhelming power: we know what can be achieved by firmness and union.[86]

The call to arms yielded quick results. Petitions and letters hostile to the infirmaries bill flowed into Dublin Castle and parliament from every quarter of the country.[87] Deputations of medical dignitaries were dispatched to London to plead with Sir John Young, the new chief secretary. The *Dublin Medical Press* continued to lash out at the Poor Law Commission. Power reacted by preparing amendments in an attempt to deflect the attacks and yet maintain the essence of the bill. But the strength of the opposition continued to mount and by the end of June the chief commissioner was forced to acknowledge in a memo to Larcom that the bill had been withdrawn.[88]

Although soundly defeated the commission was not prepared to give up on the hospital scheme. It was more than a question of administrative neatness – the desire to have all the medical charities in one organisational basket. The country's need for a comprehensive hospital system was very real. Dispensary

---

86 *DMP* xxxi (1854), 312.
87 A thick file containing these documents is in the state paper office, Dublin, CSO/OP, 1854/32.
88 Power to Larcom, 30 June 1854, Larcom Papers, MS 7780.

medical officers were faced daily with serious accident cases as well as various non-contagious ailments which ought properly to have received hospital care. Yet in many, if not most, instances the county infirmaries were too far away to be of any use. In these circumstances the Poor Law Commission and its boards of guardians collaborated in an evasion of the law. Under their control were 163 workhouse infirmaries and 146 fever hospitals. The latter were legally permitted to admit poor persons if suffering from contagious diseases while the former were limited to the treatment of workhouse inmates. But in the mid-1850s the guardians began to allow the admission of accident cases and non-contagious disease patients to both kinds of institutions and the commission winked at the practice.[89] In 1857 a first attempt was made to legalise it.

The 1854 experience had made it abundantly clear that it would be impossible to create a general hospital system based on the county infirmaries. The commission therefore prepared a bill proposing that victims of accidents and patients suffering from non-contagious diseases be allowed to enter the workhouse infirmaries for treatment. Moreover, persons considered by the guardians to be able to pay moderate fees toward their medical care would be asked to reimburse the union for the treatment, food and lodging they received. Finally, since the county infirmaries had such excellent staffs, it was proposed to allow the referral of especially difficult and complex cases to them, the costs for care and treatment being borne by the poor rate.[90]

The 1857 measure failed to reach its second reading, the incumbent government having fallen before that was possible. In the following year the new Tory chief secretary, Lord Naas, introduced a similar bill. The reaction in Ireland was far from encouraging. Landlords argued that the workhouse infirmary provisions would lead to a vast increase in the poor rates. The doctors were negative too, claiming that persons above the poverty line would be humiliated by the experience of going to a workhouse infirmary. A delegation of the Irish Medical Association met Naas in April and voiced their objections not only to the workhouse concept but to another provision which they found even more alarming, the clause that equalised the duties of the poor law inspectors thus allowing regular inspectors to perform the same tasks as the medical inspectors.[91] The *Dublin Medical Press* saw in this an attempt to eliminate the medical personnel from the upper levels of the commission and thus negate one of the major safeguards of the Medical Charities Act.

Another abortive attempt at legislation was made in 1860, but it was stopped by the same combination of forces which had halted its predecessor two years earlier. Finally, in 1862, the Poor Law (Ireland) Amendment Act

[89] *Sixteenth and eleventh annual report*, 352.

[90] *Bill to amend the laws in force for relief of the destitute poor in Ireland* (HC 1857–8, iii), 435, 447.

[91] DMP xxxix (1858), 235.

(23 & 26 Vic., c. 83) legalised the admission of poor persons with non-contagious medical problems into workhouse infirmaries. Thus was forged, in the words of the Poor Law Commission, 'the last link . . . in the connexion between the Poor Law and the older system of Medical Charities in Ireland'.[92] It had been a difficult and frustrating struggle, but nothing demonstrated the commitment of the commission to its medical responsibilities as clearly as its tenacious effort to acquire a hospital system to augment its dispensaries. The frequently expressed fears that the workhouses would be flooded with applications for free medical care proved to be unfounded. But admissions of the new categories of patients did increase significantly in the following years, vindicating the commission's arguments. In 1859 over 70,000 such patients had been treated illegally.[93] As the probability of legalisation increased so did enrolments – 76,000 in 1860, 84,000 in 1861, 98,000 in 1862, and more than 100,000 cases in 1863, the first full year of operation under the new law. That appears to have been the upper limit of demand for such services. Thereafter, admissions declined slightly and then stabilised at about 90,000 cases per year on into the following decade.[94]

With the conversion of the workhouse infirmaries into general hospitals expansion and innovation in poor law medical relief in Ireland was largely at an end. The concept of an inter-related dispensary and district hospital system, first proposed thirty years before, had now been realised. Not perhaps as its idealistic proponents had envisaged in the fullness of their dreams, but the institutional form was roughly equivalent. The Poor Law Commission was clearly pleased and concluded its 1863 report with the opinion that 'there is now probably no country which possesses a more comprehensive or better organised system of intern and extern medical relief, established and secured by law, than Ireland'.[95]

Of course by modern standards this medical care system left much to be desired. Facilities and services were less satisfactory in reality than they appeared to be on paper, especially in the poorer areas of the country. In the 1860s critics charged that the workhouse infirmaries were often unsanitary, provided inadequate diets and were understaffed.[96] In 1909 the famous Royal Commission on Poor Relief noted that

> there are many other defects, chiefly structural, in the Irish workhouse hospitals. They are for the most part the original infirmary buildings which were constructed in 1841, and except in large urban Unions have undergone little

---

92 *Sixteenth and eleventh annual report*, 352–3.
93 *Thirteenth and eighth annual report* (HC 1860, xxxvii), 530.
94 As with the data on cancellations of dispensary tickets no comprehensive tables for hospital admittances are available. But the figures for each year after 1859 are found in the statistical appendices at the end of the annual reports.
95 *Sixteenth and eleventh annual report*, 353.
96 Kelly, 'Workhouse to hospital', 51–60.

or no alteration. The wards are plain, cheerless, wholly deficient in day room accomodations and . . . ill adapted to the requirements of the sick.[97]

As the report went on to note, these conditions were largely a function of the limited financial resources available in a country as poor as Ireland. Both dispensary and workhouse medical officers were underpaid and remained so right into the twentieth century. There is no doubt that state medicine in Ireland was achieved on the cheap and a great many corners were cut in the process.

Nevertheless, allowing for all such complaints, what else could realistically have been expected? It was an inescapable fact that Ireland was poor. Even with vastly greater resources at her disposal England's record in this line was markedly less impressive until around the time of the First World War. In the context of mid nineteenth-century assumptions about property rights, taxation, the role of the state and the effectiveness of medical care, what is noteworthy is that the Irish government achieved as much as it did. Of course the Irish medical profession harped ceaselessly on the deficiencies of the dispensary and hospital systems. It was in their interest to do so. The *Dublin Medical Press* represented the profession and consistently championed its causes in every way it thought useful. Moreover, it was also its duty to set, at any given moment, the highest conceivable standards for public health. But that did not mean that the government or the country at large had to agree with or could afford the recommendations of the doctors. Indeed we might venture to consider whether or not they could have done any better if somehow they had found themselves in control of a national medical charities board, a power they courted so fervently in the 1840s. Could they have squeezed significantly greater sums out of the Irish ratepayers? Would they have worked comfortably and harmoniously with Dublin Castle? It does not seem likely. As it was the Poor Law Commission allocated a substantially greater proportion of the poor rate to medical care than did either the Scottish or English poor law authorities.

Furthermore, any division of authority between a medical charities board and the Irish Poor Law Commission would probably have produced disputes and tensions that would have reduced rather than improved the conduct of Irish medical relief; and such a division might well have deprived Ireland of perhaps the greatest single advantage she realised from the concentration of power in the commission – the surprising record achieved in epidemic control and vaccination in the 1850s and 1860s.

---

[97] *Royal Commission report*, 72–3.

6

The Medical Charities Act
and Public Health in Ireland, 1851–1872

To contemporary observers familiar with the long debate over reform of the Irish medical charities, the most important consequence of the Medical Charities Act appeared to be in the realm of the administration of medical care. But the act made important changes in the nature of public health authority as well. Virtually unnoticed was Clause 19 making the Irish Poor Law Commission the agency in Ireland for the implementation of the Nuisances Removal and Diseases Prevention Acts of 1848 and 1849 (11 & 12 Vic., c. 123 and 12 & 13 Vic., c. 111), the basic sanitary statutes then in force in the United Kingdom. This authority, formerly vested in the Irish Privy Council, had been ineffectively exercised by the Central Board of Health created during the famine emergency. Under the direction of the Poor Law Commission and augmented by subsequent and stronger laws, however, provision for state intervention in public health emergencies became more effective in Ireland in the next two decades than in any other part of the British Isles.

Medical science was still some decades away from discovering the microbiological agents that cause infectious diseases but by the 1840s many concerned observers saw a clear correlation between disease and dirt. The prevalent theory explaining the connection held that disease was generated by filth itself, or to put it more precisely, that accumulations of decomposing organic material produced an atmosphere or 'miasma' of fouled air which, when inhaled, caused the victim to sicken.[1] Edwin Chadwick and his associates at the General Board of Health were convinced of this 'miasmatic' theory. As Chadwick put it, 'All smell is, if it be intense, immediate acute disease; and eventually we may say that, by depressing the system and rendering it susceptible to the action of other causes, ALL smell is disease.'[2] Consequently, for Chadwick and other public health reformers of the 1840s and 1850s, the key to disease prevention was the enactment and enforcement of comprehensive sanitation measures, a view reflected in the provisions of the Nuisances Removal and Diseases Prevention Acts.

As applied to Ireland these statutes empowered the poor law authorities to eliminate dirt in a number of ways. Boards of guardians were given authority

---

[1] William M. Frazer, A history of English public health 1834–1939, London 1950, 38–40.
[2] Finer, Chadwick, 298.

to proceed against the owners or occupiers of property containing nuisances when they, the guardians, were notified in writing of the existence of such deposits by any two householders, or by a medical or relieving officer in the union, or by any two constables. If the persons responsible for the nuisance did not themselves remove it, the guardians could have it removed charging those persons with the costs. Moreover, if such costs could not be recovered in that fashion, they were then chargeable to the rates of the electoral division within which the nuisance occurred. Guardians were advised that nuisances located in towns or parishes or other areas which had their own local governmental authorities would probably be best left to the action of those authorities. But if they were not removed the guardians remained the agency of final responsibility and were authorised to take appropriate measures.[3] Under the Nuisances Removal and Diseases Prevention Acts each board of guardians was continuously in possession of these sanitary powers and needed no authorisation from the Poor Law Commission to use them. Unfortunately for the health of the Irish people, boards of guardians rarely possessed the vision or money to make effective use of their sanitary authority. Nor did the commission generally insist that they do so. In the 1850s and 1860s Irish cities and towns moved slowly and grudgingly away from the largely unsanitary state they had exhibited prior to the passing of the Medical Charities Act. However, when an epidemic occurred in the country, the story was somewhat different. The commission was empowered and inclined, under such circumstances, to take more extreme measures. The autumn of 1853 provided such an opportunity, for news was received in September that cholera had broken out in Newcastle-upon-Tyne.

Asiatic cholera was the most terrifying disease to afflict Europe in the nineteenth century.[4] Originating in India, where it had become epidemic in 1816, it had been unknown in Europe until the 1830s when it spread westward in the first of four great pandemics that reached as far as North America. Great Britain and Ireland were struck in 1831–2, 1848–9, 1853–4 and 1865–6. Mortality in the first two of these epidemics had been very high. England suffered almost 22,000 deaths in the first and more than 53,000 in the second. In proportion to its population Ireland had been hit even harder, 20,000 dying in 1831–2 and over 30,000 in 1848–9.[5]

Cholera is caused by a bacillis, identified by Robert Koch in 1884 as the *uibrio cholerae*, which when swallowed lodges and breeds in the intestinal

---

[3] Removal of nuisances, Circular to Boards of Guardians, *First annual report*, appendix A, no. 46, 412–15.

[4] The best discussion of the nature of cholera and the reaction to it within the English medical and scientific community in the nineteenth century is Margaret Pelling, *Cholera, fever and English medicine 1825–1865*, London 1978. I have also found useful the accounts in Finer, *Chadwick*; Frazer, *English public health*; and Anthony Wohl, *Endangered lives: public health in Victorian Britain*, London 1983.

[5] Creighton, *Epidemics in Britain*, 816, 840, 843.

tract. The most seriously affected suffer from abdominal pains, vomiting and an intense diarrhoea of a characteristic 'rice water' consistency. If not treated immediately these symptoms are often followed by a metabolic collapse in which the patient exhibits shallow breathing, weak pulse and cold, shrunken skin of a blue cast. Death can come with amazing suddenness, literally within a few hours of the onset of the illness.[6]

Cholera is transmitted from one person to another via the discharges of its victims which teem with the *vibrio*. In the crowded, filthy hovels of the agricultural labourers or in the even dirtier and more densely populated lower class slums of Victorian cities such contact was often quite direct and, given the scarcity of water for washing and the absence of modern toilet facilities, probably unavoidable. Under such circumstances the disease frequently spread through entire families in a matter of days. However, because the *vibrio* can live in water up to a fortnight, it contaminated water supplies as well. Since purification of drinking water was unthought of in this period and communities simply obtained it from the same source into which they flushed their wastes, the contagion spread through towns and cities with great rapidity. Indeed, it was this very waterborne characteristic of the disease which brought it into the homes of the middle and upper classes where personal hygiene made direct contact with the *vibrio* much less likely.

That cholera is a waterborne disease had been demonstrated as early as 1849 by Dr John Snow (1813–58), who, in a classic example of epidemiological technique, investigated each case of cholera in a London neighbourhood and traced the disease to a specific pump.[7] When he persuaded the vestry to shut it down the disease abated. Snow published his findings in 1849 but in the absence of a clear understanding of the bacteriological agents fundamentally responsible for the disease most medical authorities dismissed his theory as unsound. Nevertheless, even without knowing what precisely caused disease, the provisions of the Nuisances Removal and Diseases Prevention Acts, if carefully and thoroughly applied, could achieve positive results. The news that the disease was on the march again brought these measures into operation all over the British Isles and provided the first test for the Poor Law Commission in its new capacity as a national board of health.

Cholera appeared in Ireland in early November 1853 when outbreaks occurred simultaneously in Belfast and Cork. No sooner was it thought to be under control in those sites than it appeared in Limerick in February 1854 and in subsequent months spread into many parts of the country. The commission reacted to the epidemic with a two-stage programme consisting of general sanitary measures followed by a concentrated effort to control the disease when it made its appearance in any given locality. When cholera had

6 Finer, *Chadwick*, 333–4.
7 Frazer, *English public health*, 63. A full discussion of Snow's work, his theory of cholera propagation, and why it was not embraced immediately by the English medical community can be found in Pelling, *Cholera*, 203–49.

been reported in England in September the commission had notified its boards of guardians and issued a general order putting the special sanitary provisions of the Nuisances Removal and Diseases Prevention Acts into force throughout Ireland.[8] Under this order county surveyors, trustees and other persons responsible for the care and management of public thorough-fares were required to have all 'streets, rows, lanes, courts, alleys, and pas-sages' frequently and effectively cleaned. Moreover, when any dwelling was found to be dirty or to contain a 'foul and offensive ditch, drain, gutter, privy, cesspool, etc.', or where any swine or other animals were kept, the owner or occupier was required to 'clean, whitewash and otherwise purify' the place with all reasonable speed. The guardians were to supervise these activities and, when delays or disobedience were detected, to carry them out them-selves taking whatever steps were necessary to accomplish the goal. Such was the alarm created by the threat of cholera that the Poor Law Commission had no trouble gaining the co-operation of the local authorities and it re-ported that the guardians and sanitary committees in the towns, with few exceptions, demonstrated great zeal in carrying out these tasks. The commis-sion concluded that 'an amount of sanitary improvement has effected in this country, nothing remotely approaching to which has been ever, on any previous occasion [been] reached in a similar period'.[9]

These were simply sanitary precautions however. Once cholera actually made an appearance in a given locality much stronger measures were re-quired. In that event the Poor Law Commission issued a cholera order which mobilised the poor law apparatus, especially the dispensary system, in an all-out effort to disinfect affected areas and to isolate and treat victims of the disease.[10] Each committee of management was made a sanitary committee and every member, including the medical officers, relieving officers and war-dens were to aid the guardians in executing the emergency provisions. Medi-cal officers were designated 'medical officers for the treatment of diarrhoea and cholera' and required to give immediate aid and medicine to all persons complaining of looseness of the bowels, diarrhoea or cholera itself, even if they did not possess the usual dispensary tickets. The medical officer was to be at his dispensary daily and the guardians were instructed to post notices around the district informing the residents of his name and the location of his home and dispensary. House-to-house visitations by the medical officers and the committee men were encouraged and sometimes pressed upon the guardians by the commission. When the presence of the disease was detected the commission suggested that the home be whitewashed and the victim

[8] Removal of nuisances, General order of 20 Sept. 1853 containing directions and regulations under the Nuisances Removal and Diseases Prevention Act of 1848, section 10, and the Medical Charities Act, section 19, Second annual report, appendix A, no. 18, 306–7.

[9] Third annual report (HC 1854–5, xvi), 207.

[10] Cholera order, Second annual report, appendix A, no. 27, 325–30.

transported to a hospital if possible. This was especially necessary if the patient lacked family or friends to carry out the orders of the medical officer. Hospital accommodation was to be separate from the workhouse. Cholera wards were to be established in which the cases could be isolated. In the workhouses themselves diarrhoea watches were set up and at the first sign of the onset of the illness the patient was taken to the cholera centre.[11] In the event of death the corpse was to be removed and buried as soon possible.

It is fashionable to ridicule the attempts of nineteenth-century medicine to treat cholera. A recent article on the subject begins, 'In the whole of the history of therapeutics before the twentieth century there is no more grotesque chapter than that on the treatment of cholera, which was largely a form of benevolent homicide.'[12] While the evidence presented in this article is indisputable it is also clear that the author was unaware of the methods employed in Ireland in 1853-4. In spite of the fact that the Irish medical profession and the Poor Law Commission were completely ignorant of what causes cholera or why it kills, the treatment they proposed was sensible and may have been at least partially responsible for the comparatively low loss of life.[13]

Cholera is lethal primarily because of the rapid dehydration the victim suffers as a result of the intense vomiting and diarrhoea which deplete the body fluids and electrolytes.[14] However, if an attempt to maintain body fluids is made in the early stages of the disease, the metabolic imbalance which produces collapse and death may be averted and the patient stands a better chance of recovery. Early nineteenth-century treatments, consisting of bleeding, the use of harsh purgatives in large amounts, and the denial of water in an effort to reduce the vomiting, only accelerated the dehydration process. While bleeding was discontinued before mid-century practically everywhere, some of these other techniques were still in use for many decades. But in Ireland by 1853 the leaders of the medical profession had rejected most such 'cures' in favour of a more empirical approach based on their experience of many cholera cases in the previous two epidemics.

In a circular to its medical officers distributed in the autumn of 1853 the Poor Law Commission recommended a form of treatment based upon reports prepared both for the late Irish Central Board of Health in 1848–9 and the Irish College of Physicians in 1853. The commission observed that in nearly all cases of cholera there were two stages – the first marked by diarrhoea and the second by collapse, the so-called 'blue cholera'. The circular stressed the vital importance of immediate treatment noting that, 'All medical testimony

11 *Third annual report*, 211.
12 Norman Howard-Jones, 'Cholera therapy in the nineteenth century', *Journal of the History of Medicine* v (1972), 373.
13 Personal conversation with Dr Sarah T. Morrow, director, Guilford County Health Department.
14 Howard-Jones, 'Cholera therapy', 374.

concurs in proving that the energetic treatment of these cases had been productive of the greatest and most unquestionable benefit in checking the advances of Cholera and in saving life.'[15] It went on to state 'that when the epidemic is prevalent, mere looseness of the bowels, with or without pain, may be the commencement of the first stage of Cholera – that the disease is generally curable at this stage, and that not a moment should be lost in applying relief'. Medical officers were instructed to get patients into bed, keep them warm with hot water bottles and warm bricks, to give small quantities of whatever stimulants may be handy – brandy, whiskey, warm negus or mulled port were recommended – and to give astringent powders in warm milk after every evacuation. Most important, patients were to be allowed to drink freely 'as experience shows that denial of drink does not check vomiting while it increases very much the sufferings of the patient from the burning thirst that so often accompanies the disease'.[16]

Recommended medicines included carbonate of ammonia, a compound of powdered chalk with opium and pills of mercury and opium which contained a fourth grain of calomel (mercurous chloride), a fourth grain of opium and a fourth grain of mercury with chalk all made up with oil of caraway. While strange by modern standards, the effect of these drugs may well have been positive. Opium can have the effect of a paregoric and hence relax the bowel and slow the diarrhoea. Medical officers were specifically warned not to give castor oil or saline and other 'aperient' (laxative) substances, though in other parts of the United Kingdom the use of castor oil was advocated by well-known physicians until very late in the century.

The statistics on mortality and morbidity compiled by the Poor Law Commission in the wake of the epidemic suggested to contemporaries that these techniques had a positive effect. Of the 33,000 cases of diarrhoea reported only 5,570 advanced to the blue stage and of these only 2,606 died.[17] Compared with the mortality in England where over 24,000 fatalities were attributed to cholera in the 1853–4 epidemic, or Scotland which suffered 6,000 deaths, the Irish record was enviable.[18] The commission had worked hard to achieve it. Suggesting or even ordering procedures from Dublin was one

[15] Instructional letter regarding cholera treatment, *Second annual report*, appendix A, no. 28, 329.

[16] Extract from notification issued by the late Central Board of Health for Ireland in reference to cholera in 1848–9, ibid. no. 31, 335–6. Modern cholera treatment employs rehydration with isotonic fluids, a procedure beyond the capability of Victorian medicine. Isotonic fluids replace necessary body salts. The fluids prescribed by the IPLC in 1853 were not isotonic so that it is hard to see how the Irish treatment would have been effective with serious cases involving a substantial loss of fluid. However, moderate and slight cases might have been helped by these means.

[17] *Third annual report*, 211. There is some confusion regarding the final figure for Irish cholera fatalities in the 1853–4 epidemic. The 1856 annual report gives the total as 2,947 while the 1867 report puts it as 2,606.

[18] Creighton, *Epidemics in Britain*, 852. See also Finer, *Chadwick*, 168.

thing, having them actually carried out in the provinces was another. But the commission maintained a close watch over the execution of its directives. Weekly reports on the sanitary state of their unions were required from the guardians. Once cholera had actually been reported in a district, a medical inspector was dispatched to the spot to gather all pertinent data on the seriousness of the outbreak and its origins as well as to oversee the application of the commission's sanitation and medical relief measures.[19]

Through the spring and summer of 1854 the commission repeatedly warned the guardians against any relaxation of their efforts and even reissued the original sanitation order in September. By the end of the year the epidemic was clearly waning and early in 1855 cases were being reported only sporadically. The general order which had activated the sanitation statutes in September 1853 was allowed to expire in August 1855.

Modern medical historians reject the idea that anything Irish doctors attempted to do to mitigate the cholera in 1853–4 could have been effective. Isotonic fluids, that is those that replace salts as well as water, must be used. Clearly such treatment did not then exist. However, mortality was down substantially. Recovery of persons thought to be afflicted was frequent. From the perspective of participants it appeared that the treatment had had something to do with this result. In other words, it seemed obvious to the Poor Law Commission that the main reason Ireland had been spared the severe mortality suffered by England and Scotland, or the loss of life experienced in previous epidemics, lay in the commission's energetic application of the sanitary laws and in its control over a national network of medical personnel and facilities which could be pressed into service at very short notice. The superior organisational arrangements and the prompt and intelligent treatment provided by the poor law medical officers were thought to be the key to the recent success. The commission noted in its annual report for 1856 that the Irish people had developed confidence in the ability of the dispensary system to save them from cholera before they even knew it was among them.[20] The commission contrasted the Irish with the English experience, where the lack of a centrally directed system and adequate and timely preparation had led the local authorities to ignore the warnings of the General Board of Health until it was too late at which point they displayed 'supineness, hesitation, delay, and afterwards, panic'.[21]

In the midst of their self congratulation, however, the Poor Law Commission was brought up short by what seemed at the time a very disturbing reaction on the part of some of the guardians to the expense of the recent efforts. The duties imposed upon the medical officers by the cholera epidemic had been very heavy. In districts where the disease had been prevalent they

---

19 *Third annual report*, 210.
20 *Fourth annual report* (HC 1856, xix), 203.
21 Order issued by the Poor Law Commission to the Board of Guardians of Limerick Union, 19 Dec. 1854, ibid. appendix A, 280.

had been obliged to work long hours for many days or even weeks on end and at great risk to their own health and safety. The commission felt that substantial extra remuneration was owed to these men. The commission itself set the fees which were then to be paid by the guardians in the affected unions. Most guardians were properly reasonable, not to say grateful, and made no trouble over bonuses. The Limerick Union was an exception.

In December 1854 the Poor Law Commission ordered the Limerick guardians to pay four of their medical officers sums ranging from £40 to £90 each for cholera service.[22] The guardians refused the order, whereupon the commissioners took them to court. But the judges ruled in favour of the guardians, arguing that the statutes under which the commission operated did not give the commissioners the authority to 'value services themselves' and that to confer such a power on them would be 'monstrous'. The commissioners viewed this decision as a serious threat to their ability to mobilise the dispensary system in times of national emergency, an authority, they contended, that had been crucial to the recent success. They pointed out that if the Limerick decision was upheld in the event of subsequent epidemics they would merely have the power to inform guardians of the fact of a danger to the public health and to call on them to contract with their medical officers for treatment, a course which the commission feared would be likely to lead to the fate suffered by the General Board of Health in England.

In the event the commission's apprehensions never became reality. Although it was not until the passage of the Sanitary Act of 1866 that it received explicit authority to set medical fees for emergency service, no major epidemic occurred in the intervening years and hence no opportunity to see if a significant number of other boards of guardians would have followed Limerick's lead. It is probable that resistance of the Limerick variety was but an isolated example of local independence and stubbornness rather than the harbinger of a revolt among the guardians. The only other example of refusal to pay medical officers special fees involved the North Dublin Union in 1867 and, coming as it did after the Sanitary Act, on that occasion the Poor Law Commission won.[23] On the whole the record of co-operation between the central authority and the guardians during the cholera crisis was outstanding. Indeed, even in 1855, at the time of the quarrel with Limerick, the commission witnessed precisely contrary behaviour from the guardians of the Carrick-on-Suir Union in County Tipperary.

Scarletina (scarlet fever), a disease endemic in Ireland throughout the nineteenth century, had become epidemic in the Portlaw dispensary district in July. By September over 300 cases had been reported of which twenty-seven had died. The medical officer from the Portlaw dispensary requested

---

[22] Ibid. 206.

[23] Remuneration of medical officers in the North Dublin Union, *Twentieth and fifteenth annual report*, appendix C, V, no. 14, 589.

that the guardians provide funds for treatment and for a temporary hospital since the fever hospital at Carrick-on-Suir was six miles away, too far to transport the many patients. The guardians speedily agreed to this request. A medical inspector dispatched to the district by the Poor Law Commission reported in early October that the hospital was rapidly being established in a building secured for the purpose and that the medical arrangements were being fully and carefully carried out. By March 1856 the commission was able to report that the combination of prompt and generous action by the guardians and the skill and zeal of the medical officer had arrested the progress of the epidemic. For the commission this episode provided additional evidence of the value of the poor law medical services in Ireland as they functioned under the Medical Charities Act.[24]

The public health powers of the Poor Law Commission were not altered significantly until the Sanitary Act of 1866 (29 & 30 Vic., c. 90) was applied to Ireland. In the English context the act was a landmark measure of great importance which expanded and strengthened the powers of the Privy Council and local governmental bodies in dealing with contagious disease and nuisances. But in Ireland it made comparatively little difference. The major alteration was a shift in emphasis. In the words of John Simon (1816–1904), the medical officer to the English Privy Council who had drafted the act, 'the grammar of common sanitary legislation acquired the novel virtue of an imperative mood'.[25] In practice this meant that some of the sanitary regulations which had previously been a matter of local option were now required.

For example, guardians were to provide hospital accommodation for cholera victims as well as equipment and facilities for the disinfecting of their clothing and bedding. Daily house-to-house visitations were made mandatory, and if a sufficient number of medical officers were not available to carry out such duties, extra personnel were to be employed. The guardians were also now required to inspect and disinfect any ships (excluding those of the Royal Navy and any foreign power) found lying in waters within the boundaries of their unions just as if they were private dwellings on shore.[26] In addition it was suggested, but not required, that guardians provide shelter and support for dependants of cholera victims as was done in Liverpool.

The 1866 act also provided for an increase in the sanitary powers of local governmental bodies. In Ireland, aside from the guardians, these consisted of town councils and town commissioners. In all places where they existed they were made nuisance and sewer authorities while in all other places those powers were vested in the guardians. The powers relating to nuisances and sewers were made permanent and demanded a steady and continuous application. All three agencies were allowed to appoint inspectors for such pur-

---

[24] Correspondence on scarletina, *Fourth annual report*, appendix A, III, 267–8.
[25] Quoted in Frazer, *English public health*, 108.
[26] *Twentieth and fifteenth annual report*, 423–4.

poses and to charge their salaries to the town or borough fund or the poor rate as the case may be. In the event of epidemic, however, the Poor Law Commission was to be constituted as a national board of health responsible for all sanitary activities. Its personnel were then to carry out sanitary measures regardless of other local authorities. In other words, in times of crisis the 1866 Sanitary Act reinforced the ability of the commission to act decisively throughout the country to the exclusion of all other governmental bodies whatsoever.[27]

When cholera appeared in France and Spain in the autumn of 1865 the commission alerted the guardians to the threat and enjoined them to take appropriate action to achieve maximum cleanliness in their unions. By early July of the following year the disease was rampant in England and these warnings were reiterated. Before the month was out a case was discovered in Dublin and the commission received permission to put the sanitary acts in force throughout the country. No sooner was this done than the Sanitary Act of 1866 passed into law and came into effect in Ireland. Consequently new orders were framed consistent with its provisions. As in 1854–5 the poor law system functioned quickly and smoothly and by the end of the year the disease was fast disappearing from the island. Mortality was down slightly on the previous epidemic, amounting to 2,306 deaths, a figure which once again compared favourably with the more than 14,000 dead in England.[28]

The commission attributed this second low death toll to its unique combination of powers, facilities and personnel. At this time no other part of the United Kingdom possessed a single, central agency which could direct such a vast army of medical and other personnel to the tasks at hand. The commission became confident that it was on the way to discovering the key to epidemic control. Evidence of its sense of superiority can be gleaned from its response to advice it received from London some years later. In 1871 cholera appeared again in some of the Baltic ports creating a flurry of excitement in England. On that occasion John Simon, then the medical officer to the newly created English Local Government Board, saw fit to send certain circulars and notices which he had prepared relating to cholera prevention and control to the chief secretary's office in Ireland. Simon suggested procedures he felt should be followed in the event the disease moved westward as it had done in the past. He inquired further whether the circulars should not be sent to the various local bodies responsible for nuisances control in Ireland. Thomas Burke (1825–82), the new under-secretary (Larcom had retired in 1869), dispatched this correspondence to the Poor Law Commission for its opinion. Power replied promptly, dismissing Simon's suggestions and noting that in Ireland many of these things 'have been conducted more systemati-

---

[27] Ibid. 562–3.

[28] Ibid. 427–8. For English death totals see Creighton, *Epidemics in Britain*, 852. Proportionally England and Wales suffered 6.5 cholera deaths for every 10,000 persons and Ireland only 4.2.

cally for many years past than in Great Britain'.[29] As it turned out the disease confined itself to Scandinavia and no emergency measures were necessary in the UK. But the occasion illustrated that the Irish authorities felt they needed no lessons from even so distinguished a public health figure as John Simon. Furthermore, by 1871 the commission had further reason for thinking itself more able in these matters than their English counterparts. A comparison of the records compiled by each nation in the matter of smallpox control showed that an impressive superiority had been achieved in Ireland.

In the first half of the nineteenth century smallpox was the only serious contagious disease for which a proven preventive process had been developed – Edward Jenner's vaccination technique. But before the advent of the poor law Ireland possessed no organised system of vaccination. The Cow Pock Institute had been founded in Dublin in 1804 to collect and distribute smallpox vaccine, but for many years its operations were confined to the city and its environs.[30] Whatever vaccination was performed throughout the country was done either for a fee or as charity among the poor by doctors acting on their own initiative. But by the late 1830s frustration with the inadequacies of vaccination in England led to reform of the Irish situation as well. In 1838 the English Provincial Medical and Surgical Association in collaboration with the Medical Society of London petitioned the government for a ban on inoculation and provision of free public vaccination for the poor.[31] By 1841 parliament responded by making inoculation illegal and establishing a system of free vaccination for everyone who requested it. This was to be administered through the boards of guardians. The Vaccination Extension Act (3 & 4 Vic., c. 29) applied the system to Ireland as well.

Entrusting the process to the poor law authorities, although probably an improvement over voluntary vaccination, was not found to work as well as had been hoped. Medical men in both countries deeply resented the contract system under which their services were retained. The Irish doctors in particular were insulted by the requirement that they accept less payment than their English counterparts – 1s. for the first 200 cases, as compared to the rate of 1s. 6d., and only 6d. for every vaccination over 200. Moreover, the prospect of free vaccination was less attractive to the public than had been thought. The Irish peasants were particularly apathetic and stirred themselves to take advantage of the service only when frightened by the outbreak of smallpox in their localities.[32]

In 1851 the Medical Charities Act ended the contract system in Ireland

[29] Power to Burke, CSO/RP, 1871/17323.

[30] Fleetwood, *History of medicine*, 168–9.

[31] Lambert, 'Victorian national health service', 3.

[32] The complaints of the Irish doctors regarding the vaccination programme fill the pages of the *DMP* in the 1840s as well as those of testimony before the select committees of 1843 and 1846. See especially the testimony of William Kidd and Henry Maunsell, *Select committee* (1843), 98, 284.

and required instead that the dispensary medical officers vaccinate, free of charge, all persons who applied for it at the dispensaries. As in the past the service was not limited to the poor since no dispensary tickets were necessary. In the course of the next few years it was discovered, however, that these arrangements were not satisfactory either. Several different kinds of problems were encountered. First the medical officers received no extra payment for successful vaccinations as they had under the 1840 act. Already overworked and underpaid (at least in their own estimation) they knew that it made no financial sense for them to go out of their way to encourage free vaccination. Many, of course, were dedicated men who made the effort anyway, but the pattern that emerged in the early 1850s was one of great variation in the numbers of vaccinations from one dispensary district to another.[33] The lack of enthusiasm on the part of the doctors was exceeded only by that of their potential patients. In 1856 Dr John Hill, one of the medical inspectors, reported on the operation of the vaccination procedures under the Medical Charities Act. He claimed that there was an almost universal reluctance of the people to bring their children to the dispensaries for vaccination because of their fear of contagion through exposure to other sick people there. Furthermore, the farm labourers who constituted the bulk of the Irish population professed not to like to have vaccination performed either in the heat of the summer or in the cold of the winter. But in both the spring and the autumn they claimed to be too busy with the planting and the harvesting to find the time to bring in the children.[34]

For those parents who did get their children vaccinated another difficulty arose. They frequently failed to bring the children back for the customary eight-day check-up to see if the vaccination had taken, owing to their fear of having the vesicle punctured and the lymph drawn off, a common practice among provincial vaccinators as it allowed them to maintain a stock of fresh vaccine with which to vaccinate new patients. These people professed to believe that removal of lymph impaired or destroyed the protective power of the vaccination.[35] Hill claimed that in many districts scarcely a third of the number vaccinated were brought back for inspection, and that of these the majority had failed. Consequently the medical officers were unable to ascertain the success or failure of most of the vaccinations they performed and, in addition, they were constantly short of fresh lymph, making it necessary for them to make frequent application to the Cow Pock Institute. Even worse,

---

[33] *Second annual report* (HC 1854, xx), 224.

[34] Report from Dr John Hill, medical inspector, on gratuitous vaccination under the Medical Charities Act, *Fourth annual report*, appendix A, VI, 272–5. Hill's report constitued a seminal analysis of the problems afflicting the vaccination program in the mid-fifties. He recommended a number of reforms such as compulsory vaccination, registration of births and vaccination fees for the medical officers, all of which became Poor Law Commission policy in 1856.

[35] Ibid.

vaccination itself was brought into disrepute by the continued occurrence of smallpox in persons thought to have been protected. It was this phenomenon which continuously reinforced the faith of the tradition-steeped Irish peasantry in the other, older form of protection against smallpox, inoculation.

Inoculation was introduced into the British Isles from the Ottoman Empire by Lady Mary Wortley Montagu in the early eighteenth century.[36] Unlike vaccination, which used the harmless cowpox vaccine, inoculation used lymph from smallpox itself. Ideally an attempt was made to obtain the lymph from a person known to have suffered a mild case of the disease and to dry it for a few days in order to acquire a weakened form. Nevertheless, inoculation often resulted in considerable danger both to the individuals directly involved and to the community in which they lived. In effect the patient was given a mild form of smallpox, but in order to provide immunity the disease had to run its course. In spite of all calculation it might prove more virulent than intended and kill the patient. Moreover, whether it did or not, the patient himself became a source of contagion which could spread throughout the region. Hence inoculation could and did result in the propagation of smallpox epidemics. For that reason it had come into disrepute among medical men once Jenner's much safer technique had been clearly demonstrated in the early nineteenth century.

In spite of the warnings of the medical community, the appeals of clergy, or the penalties of the law (under the Vaccination Act inoculators could be sentenced to a month in prison), a strong prejudice in favour of inoculation existed in the minds of the Irish peasantry in the 1850s and 1860s. Inoculators were peasants themselves and hence closer to the people than the doctors, the constabulary, or the other authorities. Conviction of such men was very difficult because they were shielded by the people who hated to be forced to testify against them. To do so was apparently to be thought an informer, 'the most disgraceful character that can be, in their [the peoples'] opinion', noted one medical officer.[37] Medical officers who attempted to prosecute the inoculators were even known to have been threatened by local residents. Moreover, the inoculators could be very clever. The technique of one was described by the same medical officer in a letter to the commission in the summer of 1858. The inoculator apparently carried on a flourishing business and escaped detection in an ingenious way.

He goes to a friend's house at some distance from his own, and this is made known to the neighbourhood. A woman bringing her child to be cut, hands it to a strange woman who stands at the door; she takes it in and returns it to the woman after being inoculated, so that she can never say who did it. He never

---

36 Charles Singer and E. Ashworth Underwood, A short history of medicine, 2nd edn, New York–Oxford 1967, 199–200.

37 Correspondence on vaccination, letter from Dr W. E. Donelan, medical officer, Dunmore Dispensary, Tuam Union, Seventh annual report, appendix A, II, 370.

takes money but is always paid in kind; and he never cuts with a lancet, thinking these things save him from prosecution. One thing is certain, he escaped at Milltown, as no one could prove who inoculated the child.[38]

Occasionally inoculation could backfire on its practitioners. Dr William Geary, a poor law medical inspector, investigated such a case in Roundstone Dispensary District in County Galway in the fall of 1858. It seemed that a notorious old inoculator known as Mulroony, who was reputed to evade the authorites by going about in women's clothing, had inoculated over 300 children of whom more than twenty had died by the end of October. Geary reported that the residents had been so frightened by the epidemic that their prejudices vanished and a sudden confidence in the protection afforded by vaccination caused over 400 entries in the vaccination register in the last three weeks of October. 'Such a crowd showed up today', he reported on 1 November 'that two policemen were needed to keep order and expedite the medical officer's labours'. Nearly 200 persons were vaccinated and he commented that, 'It was gratifying to observe the readiness with which parents allowed lymph to be taken from the arms of unsuccessful cases, providing an unlimited supply.'[39] But such triumphs were momentary and isolated.

By the mid-fifties the Poor Law Commission was beginning to understand the nature of the problems associated with the vaccination programme. The annual reports increasingly register their growing concern and frustration with the failure of existing laws and arrangements to work effectively. As early as 1853 the commissioners had noted the reluctance of the Irish poor to avail themselves of the vaccination service and their preference for inoculation. Assuming this was a function of ignorance they launched an advertising campaign on the dispensary level posting notices around the districts announcing the virtues of free vaccination and stressing the danger and illegality of inoculation.[40] But instead of the anticipated improvement the number of vaccinations recorded annually actually declined. By 1856 the commissioners were becoming alarmed. Assuming a population of approximately 6,500,000 (the 1851 census figure) they calculated that there should have been about 218,000 births in 1855. Subtracting one-third for infant mortality, about 146,000 should ideally have been vaccinated under the free programme. Instead slightly fewer than 47,000 vaccinations had actually been performed, and that figure constituted a reduction of 6,000 from the previous year.[41] So much for advertising.

The commission was now convinced that only much stronger measures would suffice. In 1853 parliament had passed with little debate or apparent interest an act requiring that in England and Wales all infants were to be

38 Ibid.
39 Report of Dr Geary on the Roundstone Dispensary District, ibid. 373–4.
40 *Second annual report*, 225.
41 *Fourth annual report*, 197.

vaccinated within three months of their births.[42] Parents were to be notified of the law by the local registrar of births and deaths who also made a record of and reported the vaccinations. Failure to comply left the parents liable to legal action. Costs of the programme were borne by the poor law guardians who, as in the past, contracted with local practitioners to perform the service. The Poor Law Commission requested that the compulsory aspect of this measure and an act establishing state registration of births, deaths and marriages, without which the law was unenforceable, be extended to Ireland. Simple enough on the surface, this request ran into the inevitable Irish complications.

Civil registration of births, deaths and marriages had been in effect in England and Wales since 1836 and Scotland since 1854. But proposals to introduce it in Ireland had foundered thus far on the rock of Ireland's special religious problems. The Catholic clergy, forbidden by law to celebrate mixed marriages, were unalterably opposed.[43] Moreover, the idea of compulsory vaccination itself was opposed by some Irish MPs who did not think it fair to impose penalties on parents who did not agree to have their children vaccinated. Some argued that such compulsion would backfire and drive peasants more forcefully into the arms of the inoculators. Under these circumstances the best the commission could manage was a modest improvement in the vaccination law put forward by Lord Naas in 1858. Entitled 'An Act to make further provision for the Practice of Vaccination in Ireland' (21 & 22 Vic., c. 64) it was a far cry from what the commissioners really wanted but it did allow for some intelligent changes.

The major provisions of the act were quite straightforward.[44] Medical officers were to be paid a pound for every twenty successful vaccinations. Dispensary districts were to be subdivided into vaccination districts each of which was to contain a vaccination station located out in the countryside away from the dispensaries themselves. The stations were to be so placed as to make them convenient for the bulk of the farm labourers. Separating the vaccination centres from the dispensaries also reduced the problem of contagion often raised as an excuse, and a valid one, for failure to bring children in in the past. In addition the Poor Law Commission, demonstrating remarkable sensitivity to the rhythms of the peasants' lives and their well known wishes regarding appropriate seasons for vaccination, recommended that the medical officers visit each vaccination station at regular and frequent intervals in the spring and autumn when the demands of planting and harvest made visits to the dispensaries especially difficult. The act also facilitated the effort to eliminate inoculators by allowing the costs of their prosecution to be defrayed out of the rates. Most boards of guardians responded immediately to

---

42 Lambert, 'Victorian national health service', 3.
43 *Hansard*, clxix (1863), 1390.
44 Vaccination under 21 & 22 Vic., c. 64, *Seventh annual report*, appendix A, 358.

the commission's request to create vaccination districts. Those which failed to do so were ordered to comply.[45] By the spring of 1860 the reorganisation was complete. Counting the dispensaries themselves there were then 2,298 vaccination centres distributed uniformly over the country. Each spring and autumn before the medical officers were due to visit the centres the country-side around each of them was posted with the days, hours and places where free vaccination was to be made available.[46]

The initial results were encouraging. The total successful vaccinations, which had reached 47,855 in 1857 and 54,984 in 1858, ballooned to 140,411 in 1859, the first full year under the new arrangements. But the commission was not deceived into thinking that this considerable improvement meant that their troubles were over. Nor were they convinced that the recent vaccination act had achieved or would achieve the level of vaccination they thought appropriate for the island. This scepticism was based on careful scrutiny of the record of each medical officer in each vaccination district in the country; a detailed survey which revealed what the raw total did not – a continued and widespread variance in performance.[47] Moreover, as the *Dublin Medical Press* pointed out, one could not be sure that the figures turned in by the medical officers actually indicated successful vaccinations as distinct from vaccinations performed.[48] If parents failed to bring their children back to be checked it was asking a great deal of the vaccinator not to report such cases as successful anyway, since if he did not he would receive no payment for them. Overworked and underpaid medical officers must have succumbed to this temptation frequently. The commission, therefore, viewed the recent vaccination act and the increase in reported vaccinations as a gratifying improvement but not a permanent solution. They continued to press for the English system of compulsory vaccination in combination with birth registration.

Over the next few years the vaccination statistics bore out both the commission's insight and its fears. The 140,411 vaccinations in 1859 declined to 107,305 in 1860 and then to 90,256 the following year.[49] In spite of an increase in 1862 these figures revealed the failure of the voluntary system. In 1863, therefore, with the *Dublin Medical Press*, the Irish Medical Association and the government solidly behind him, Sir Robert Peel (1822–95), eldest son of the distinguished Tory prime minister and from 1861 to 1865 chief secretary for Ireland, at last guided through parliament the legislation the commission desired.[50]

Bills for the registration of births and deaths and for compulsory vaccina-

---

45 Ibid.
46 *Thirteenth and eighth annual report* (HC 1860, xxxvii), 346.
47 Ibid. 348–51.
48 *DMP* ns ii (1860), 403–4.
49 *Fifteenth and tenth annual report*, 560.
50 *DMP* ns vii (1863), 327, 568.

tion were presented to the House of Commons as separate measures. Peel had surprisingly little trouble getting them through. He avoided the problem of religion by confining the measure to births and deaths, simply leaving out registration of marriages.[51] When some Irish members objected and raised the old questions Peel dismissed their charges as irrelevant to his measures and marshalled the votes to beat down an amendment designed to include mar- riage registration and thus sink the whole package. Defeated on that front, opponents raised the familiar cry of poverty, arguing that Irish ratepayers were already overburdened and that the additional costs of the new pro- gramme should be taken out of the consolidated fund. But Peel argued that the costs were paltry and that since English and Scottish ratepayers were forced to bear them it was impossible to grant special privileges to their Irish counterparts.[52] Nor did the argument that compulsory vaccination would increase inoculation in Ireland, rather than decrease it as intended, gain any significant support. As usual attendance of Irish members at the late night sessions when the Commons invariably debated these measures was slight. The government was obviously intent on getting them through and, backed by solid majorities, they moved easily through both houses and came into effect on 1 January 1864.

The Births and Deaths Registration (Ireland) Act (26 & 27 Vic., c. 11) and the Compulsory Vaccination (Ireland) Act (26 & 27 Vic., c. 52) rapidly proved to be much more effective in Ireland than similar measures had been in other parts of the United Kingdom. The primary reason appeared to be the Irish dispensary system. As in the past medical officers continued to be the public vaccinators, but they were to be births and deaths registrars as well. Combining both functions was not mandatory, but in fact virtually all the medical officers leapt at the opportunity because of the fees, 1s. for every birth and death.[53] In sparsely populated regions the medical officers could not afford to pass up the money.

But their need worked to make the new legislation effective. As both registrars and vaccinators the dispensary medical officers were in a unique position to oversee and promote the vaccination programme. As registrar the medical officer was informed of all births in the district and used the occasion to serve the new parents with a notice informing them of the law and requiring them to present their child for vaccination within six months of its birth. Failure to comply required the medical officer to inform the guardians who were then expected to prosecute. Conviction brought a maximum fine of 10s., a stiff penalty for the poor.

The Poor Law Commission understood that the key to the effectiveness of the compulsory programme lay in the willingness of the guardians and magis-

---

[51] *Hansard*, clxix (1863), 612–22.
[52] Ibid. clxx (1863), 651–2.
[53] Circulars to Boards of Guardians on the Compulsory Vaccination Act, *Seventeenth and twelfth annual report*, appendix C, II, 551–4.

trates to penalise the defaulters. If the act was not enforced on the local level it would be no better than the voluntary system. Consequently, the commission paid very close attention to the proceedings of the guardians, even going so far as to maintain a weekly supervision of their meetings. 'Under this practice', the commissioners commented in 1868, 'we omitted no opportunity of impressing upon the Guardians their duty to enforce a law made for the protection of helpless children.'[54] Although they encountered unwillingness to convict defaulters in some unions, on the whole the act was remarkably effective.

In 1864, the first full year of operation, almost 192,000 persons were vaccinated, nearly double the figure for the previous year. This exceptional increase was due to a fortunate confusion which ballooned the vaccination totals well beyond what could have been expected from the annual birthrate. Technically the act applied only to children born after 31 December 1863. But the Irish peasants failed to grasp this detail and, fearing prosecution, brought in their older children as well.[55] In subsequent years total vaccinations declined to less impressive levels but never fell below 125,000 in the next decade, an indication of how many children had been missed by the voluntary programme.

The effectiveness of the compulsory system was rapidly revealed in the dramatic improvement in the mortality statistics for smallpox in the years after 1864. Heretofore, smallpox had been a major killer in Ireland. Over 7,000 deaths were attributed to it in 1838 alone, and the average mortality in that decade was nearly 6,000 deaths per year.[56] In the 1840s things were little better with a high of 6,436 deaths in 1849 and a low of 2,453 five years earlier. The improved economic conditions in the post-famine period, combined with the first serious efforts to combat smallpox, had doubtlessly contributed to the comparatively low annual rate of about 1,700 deaths in the 1850s. But that reduction hardly prepared the commission for the drop to statistically insignificant levels in the late sixties. In the four years 1867–70 only 338 cases of the disease were recorded of which ninety-nine died, an average of twenty-five per year.[57]

None the less the Poor Law Commission was not satisfied. Their concern was more than merely bureaucratic tidiness. Of the ninety-nine deaths recorded in 1867–70, sixty-seven had occurred in a two-week period in 1868 and were directly traceable to the work of a single inoculator.[58] The commissioners blamed both the local guardians and the magistrates, the former

54 *Twenty-first and sixteenth annual report*, 445.
55 *Eighteenth and thirteenth annual report* (HC 1865, xxii), 363–5.
56 Creighton, *Epidemics in Britain*, 603, 620–1. See also *Twenty-first and sixteenth annual report*, 443, which provides a compilation of annual smallpox deaths in Ireland from the late 1830s through 1867.
57 These figures are drawn from the Poor Law Commission annual reports for 1868–71.
58 *Twenty-second and seventeenth annual report*, 377.

because they had failed to prosecute a great number of defaulting parents in their districts and the latter because of their leniency in dealing with the few brought before them. The commission rebuked the guardians, brought the conduct of the magistrates to the attention of the government, and appointed a second medical officer to the district. However, greater disappointments were in store for them.

From 1870 to 1873 the most lethal smallpox epidemic of the century raged throughout Europe. In England and Wales, where vaccination had been compulsory since 1853, over 23,000 persons succumbed to the disease in 1871 alone; and by the time the epidemic had run its course in the spring of 1873, a total of more than 44,000 deaths had been attributed to it.[59] In spite of its impressive progress in fighting the disease Ireland was not spared. Intercourse between the two countries was constant and heavy and quarantine regulations were vague and ineffectually applied. Hence smallpox victims poured into Ireland in 1870 and 1871 when the epidemic was getting under way in England.

The Poor Law Commission insisted that the guardians whose unions bordered on the east coast and contained harbours must provide hospital accommodation for the treatment and isolation of victims. A major outbreak occurred in Belfast in 1871 and the full dispensary and hospital facilities of the poor law administration were thrown into action to halt the spread of infection. Extra accommodation was prepared in workhouse infirmaries and fever hospitals. When persons refused to go to hospital medical officers were instructed to disinfect their houses and vaccinate and revaccinate all local residents.[60]

These precautions appeared to work reasonably well in 1871 and the death total of 647, though high in comparison to the years immediately preceding it, was very low when compared to that of England. Yet smallpox had gained a foothold in the country. Many persons who had never been vaccinated or who had been vaccinated many years earlier as children, were susceptible to this particularly virulent form of the disease. Consequently 1872 was a terrible year with over 10,000 cases of smallpox of which over 3,000 died. Subsequently the epidemic waned. The following year brought a death toll of 481.

The great smallpox epidemic notwithstanding, the Poor Law Commission looked upon the twenty years following the passage of the Medical Charities Act as a period during which it had demonstrated the value of its form of state medicine. While it had devoted most of its attention to reducing the ravages of cholera and smallpox the incidence of other contagious diseases had declined as well. Most noteworthy was the reduction in typhus and other

[59] Creighton, *Epidemics in Britain*, 614–16, 620. See also Brand, *Doctors and the state*, 46–7.
[60] *Twenty-fifth and twentieth annual report*, 34.

forms of fever which had been routinely epidemic in Ireland for as far back as one cared to look. By the mid-1860s it had become evident to all observers that the devastating fever epidemics which had been a feature of every decade before mid-century were now a thing of the past. The failure of the potato in Connaught and Munster in the early sixties had produced what the Poor Law Commission referred to as an 'epidemic constitution', but no epidemic had resulted. They attributed this non-event largely to the vastly improved standard of living consequent on economic expansion and continued emigration in the wake of the massive population reductions of the famine years. But they also felt the availability of medical care through the dispensaries and the capacity to isolate fever victims in the fever hospitals had played an important role in bringing the old Irish plague under control.[61]

By 1872 state medicine, as it was understood by the commission, was firmly established in Ireland. The controversy over reform and control of the medical charities which had punctuated the 1830s and 1840s had gradually subsided in the face of the commission's success in the 1850s and 1860s. In the process a hodge-podge of largely unorganised, unsupervised and unco-ordinated medical facilities had been welded into a rationally administered, nationwide system providing the Irish poor with the most comprehensive free medical care available in the British Isles. At the same time the value of the dispensary system for epidemic control and vaccination had been amply demonstrated.

Doubtless the system looked better from the vantage point of Customs House than from the dispensaries themselves, and better then than it does now given our more accurate notions about the nature of disease and the scant likelihood that mid nineteenth-century medicine could do anything important for its patients. Indeed, well into the present century critics harped ceaselessly on the penuriousness of the poor law approach to medical relief. Moreover, the centralised and bureaucratic nature of the system undoubtedly produced a rigidity which affected both patients and personnel. The former had to accept whatever the local medical officer felt appropriate by way of treatment and care while the medical officers themselves never ceased to feel exploited both by the guardians and the central authority.

None the less, in spite of its warts, the fact that both the conception and the realisation of state medicine had been carried so far in Ireland by the 1870s was the crucial achievement. It is noteworthy that the conception had been formulated so clearly and so early. The simultaneous proposals for a national health service made by Dr Phelan and the Poor Inquiry Commission in the mid-1830s had set the standard against which all subsequent plans were judged. Realisation of their ideas had been marked by thirty years of contention and compromise and remained far from complete. But in the

---

[61] *Twenty-first and sixteenth annual report*, 427–30. This report contains an extensive discussion of Irish fever epidemics in the eighteenth and early nineteenth centuries.

interval a significant and unique form of state health service had been developed which, regardless of its financial and technical deficiences, represented the government's acknowledgment of a basic responsibility for the health of its poorer citizens.

Moreover, the success of the Irish dispensary system had implications for the development of state medicine in England for it furnished evidence of the feasibility of such a programme at a time when the English administrators and public felt free medical care socially demoralising and financially irresponsible. Although it would be many years before the English government would be willing to commit itself wholeheartedly to such programmes, the Irish experience began to affect English public health policy and administration in the 1860s and contributed to that gradual change in official and public opinion which eventually made a state health service acceptable in the larger and more urbanised nation.

7

The Irish Dispensary System and Reform in England, 1866–1876

Historians of the English poor law now see the 1860s as a turbulent period out of which emerged a strengthened institution more fully in line with the vision of 1834. As M. E. Rose puts it 'by the mid-1870s, the English Poor Law had come through its decade of crisis and had been so reconstructed as to be within sight of realising the Chadwickian ideal'.[1] This 'decade of crisis' had involved virtually all aspects of the poor law authority's brief. Of particular moment – for several years claiming centre stage – was a protracted debate over poor law medical relief. In addition, though not at the time part of the Poor Law Board's central responsibilities, matters relating to the nation's public health also came in for close scrutiny and excited many to clamour for a major effort at reform. In this context the forms of medical relief and epidemic control which had been developed in Ireland since 1851 began to attract the attention both of English medical reformers and of the English Poor Law Board itself.

At mid-century England provided medical care for the poor through a mixed system of public and private charity. The former in the shape of poor law medical relief; the latter via a complex variety of medical charities and self-help institutions. The most important and numerous charities were the voluntary hospitals and public dispensaries. The voluntary hospitals, concentrated in London and the larger provincial towns, treated the sick poor recommended to them by subscribers and personnel authorised to distribute tickets. The public dispensaries were frequently associated with the voluntary hospitals serving as outpatient centres and resembled them in their dependence on charitable gifts and subscriptions, the fact that they made no charge for their treatment and medicines, and that the medical personnel donated their services. By mid-century public dispensaries were very widespread, having been established in virtually every town in the country.[2]

The self-help institutions consisted largely of medical clubs and provident dispensaries. They had grown substantially as a result of the initial tightening of poor law medical charity in the reorganisation resulting from the adoption

---

[1] M. E. Rose, 'The crisis of poor relief in England 1860–1890', in W. J. Mommsen (ed.) with Wolfgang Mock, *The emergence of the welfare state in Britain and Germany 1850–1950*, London 1981, 62.

[2] Hodgkinson, *Origins*, 185–214, 592–602, 610–12. See also Woodward, *To do the sick no harm*, 36–60, and Abel-Smith, *Hospitals*, ch. iii.

of the new poor law in 1834. Since the new poor law had originally been focused on paupers, and able-bodied paupers at that, persons somewhat above the poverty line, who had heretofore often received care under the old poor law arrangements, turned to the self-help agencies as a kind of health insurance. Both required contributions from members and were encouraged by the poor law authorities because they were thought to stimulate independence and self-reliance among the working classes.[3] Both the medical clubs and provident dispensaries required payment from their patients. On the whole this usually took the form of subscriptions although some dispensaries were fortunate enough to receive charitable gifts as well. Overall the provident dispensaries appear to have worked rather better than did the clubs. Many provided death benefits and disability income as well as medical care and were noted for the quality of their drugs and treatment.[4]

However, in spite of its growth and obvious benefit to the poor, private medical charity was experiencing serious problems in England by mid-century. Public dispensaries were accused of being remiss in failing to screen out paupers and in not concentrating on the non-indigent patients they were intended to serve.[5] Such criticism lauded the self-help characteristic of the medical clubs and provident dispensaries but both of these institutions experienced difficulties as well. The clubs were attacked both by disgruntled members and by the medical profession. The former charged that they were not provided with adequate care or medicine and the latter accused the poor law authorities of manipulating the clubs to their own purpose. Many clubs were subsidised by guardians and the club doctor often did double duty as the poor law medical officer.

The complaints had substantial basis in fact. Forced to operate on subscriptions alone, the clubs were in constant financial trouble and as early as the 1840s were failing in many parts of the country. Though the provident dispensaries appear to have fared better than the clubs, both institutions suffered from the requirement that patients pay some part of the costs of their care. In spite of the very low subscription rates, the availability of free medicine and treatment through the voluntary hospitals, public dispensaries and the poor law system were an irresistible draw for increasing numbers of poor (and not so poor).[6] Under such circumstances some form of non-pauperising system which could be controlled and directed by the state and which involved a commitment to a formal policy rather than a haphazard, de facto, state of affairs, began to recommend itself to thoughtful observers. And the evolution

---

3   Hodgkinson, Origins, 215–49.
4   Ibid. 243.
5   Ibid. 212.
6   Lancet, 1870, i. 775. See also the correspondence between Dr Joseph Rogers and Dr Toler Maunsell on the question of provident dispensaries, British Medical Journal, 20 Jan. 1872.

of poor law medical relief suggested that the time was perhaps approaching when a coherent system might be housed within the poor law authority.

Indeed, the poor law provision of free medical charity was growing in importance by mid-century. Under the arrangements and ideas of 1834 provision of medical relief was originally incidental to ordinary poor relief and was not conceived as an important element of the new poor law programme. No medical commissioner was appointed to the Poor Law Commission, nor were there any medical inspectors, separate medical facilities, or a specific line in the budget for drugs and equipment.[7] In fact such supplies had to be provided out of the salaries of the poor law medical officers. Relief was confined to paupers and was both indoor and outdoor. Indoor relief was originally reserved for inmates of the workhouses while outdoor was determined by the relieving officer who decided if applicants were poor enough to qualify.

Experience gradually revealed to the guardians that the bulk of poor relief involved sick, aged, orphaned, widowed or deranged people rather than able-bodied adults. Moreover, the effort to enforce a policy of indoor relief as the general rule broke down in the face of fierce resistance, especially in the north of England. Consequently, significant deviations from the recommendations of the 1834 report occurred throughout the country. Recognising the need to provide some care for the sick, guardians hired medical officers as a matter of course in the period of reorganisation in the late thirties. The General Medical Order of 1842 gave official sanction to the poor law medical service, regularised the size of medical districts, and improved service for chronic cases. An additional change occurred in 1852 when the Poor Law Board authorised guardians to provide medical relief in instances where the head of the family was still employed as long as it could be determined that he could not afford to pay for medical treatment. In the same decade workhouse infirmaries were opened to persons not receiving ordinary indoor relief. Hence, in the 1850s and 1860s workhouses increasingly came to resemble public hospitals rather than merely sick wards of union workhouses.[8]

Although these changes increased the medical role of the poor law and hinted at the much greater changes shortly to come, their impact should not be over-estimated. The new regulations were permissive rather than obligatory and therefore unevenly applied. On the whole boards of guardians were more committed to a tight-fisted policy of less eligibility on all levels of relief than was the central authority. Furthermore, guardians in England could not be coerced by the Poor Law Board as readily as in Ireland and were likely to do as they pleased. This comparatively restrictive approach to medical relief is reflected in the annual expenditures. From 1849 to 1867 the proportion of the poor law budget devoted to medical relief in England and Wales ranged

[7] Hodgkinson, Origins, 73–5, 120–1. See also Sidney Webb and Beatrice Webb, English local government, X: English poor law policy, 8.
[8] Hodgkinson, Origins, 451; Fraser, British welfare state, 84–5.

from 3.6 per cent to 4.2 per cent of the total.[9] In Ireland expenditures on the dispensary system alone accounted for between 10 and 19 per cent for the period 1853–67.[10]

Finally, for many critics the worst feature of English poor law medical relief was the fact that the infirmaries were generally located within mixed workhouses where patients were brought into contact with the deranged and the dissolute. Merely changing admissions policies, it was charged, was not likely to encourage broader use under such circumstances. The system was therefore far from satisfactory in the view of many observers and increasingly attracted critical attention. Reform-minded men and women, many of them well-connected socially and politically, began to create organisations through which their concerns could be articulated. One such was the National Association for the Promotion of Social Science, founded in the late 1850s with the aim of improving knowledge regarding the whole range of social problems confronting the country. Another was the Workhouse Visiting Society, whose special focus was the increasingly unsatisfactory nature of poor law workhouse care. Both of these bodies made use of the press to publicise their concerns.[11] Consequently, by the mid-sixties, awareness of serious inadequacies in poor law medical care had become widespread and a single incident was sufficient to trigger a major reform effort.

In December 1864 the *Times* accused the Poor Law Board of gross negligence in the death of a pauper in the Holborn workhouse infirmary.[12] A second death in another London workhouse a few weeks later further strengthened the position of those critical of the poor law and initiated a full-scale attack on the medical policy of the Poor Law Board. Playing a major role in the demand for an inquiry was Florence Nightingale, the heroine of the Scutari hospital wards in the Crimean War a decade earlier. Since her return Miss Nightingale had devoted herself to various efforts at medical reform in England, first in the War Department and subsequently in the field of nursing which she was fast turning into a respectable profession for middle-class women.[13] In the mid-sixties she was actively involved in organising and training nurses for work in the poor law infirmaries. A woman of extraordinary energy and will, she tended to dominate those with whom she came into contact, including cabinet ministers, even though she was by this time an invalid who seldom ventured beyond her hotel room.[14]

9 Hodgkinson, *Origins*, 296, table 11.3.
10 *Twentieth and fifteenth report*, 416.
11 Abel-Smith, *Hospitals*, 70–1.
12 Gwendoline Ayers, *England's first state hospitals and the Metropolitan Asylums Board 1867–1930*, Berkeley–Los Angeles 1971, 6.
13 The standard account remains Edward Cook, *The life of Florence Nightingale*, London 1913. See also Cecil Woodham-Smith, *Florence Nightingale, 1820–1910*, London 1950, and F. B. Smith, *Florence Nightingale*, New York 1982.
14 Woodham-Smith, *Florence Nightingale*, 215–16.

Already well-informed about the sad state of the workhouses, Miss Nightingale used the occasion of the *Times* attack to press for major reforms. Her influence secured an interview with the Liberal president of the Poor Law Board, Charles Villiers, who promptly fell under her spell. Villiers ordered an investigation of every workhouse infirmary and sick ward in London. His internal effort was further stimulated by an outside inquiry begun by the *Lancet* in the summer of 1865.[15] For fully a year and a half the medical journal printed detailed and overwhelmingly critical accounts of the condition of poor law medical facilities and services in the metropolis. At its annual conference in the same year, the British Medical Association pledged support for the *Lancet's* efforts and instituted a further inquiry of its own.[16] By 1866 the agitation was rapidly becoming a movement for reform and was attracting broad public support, including that of eminent laymen like Charles Dickens and John Stuart Mill.

Upon the change in government in June 1866, Villiers was replaced at the Poor Law Board by the Conservative Gathorne Hardy. Miss Nightingale, now working in concert with her friend and ally in sanitary reform matters, Edwin Chadwick, immediately sought to win the same influence with the new president that she had come to exercise over his predecessor.[17] Gathorne Hardy was not susceptible to the Nightingale charm, however. He thanked her politely for her interest in workhouse infirmary reform, declined an invitation to hear her views at couchside, and ignored her repeated letters and appeals. The issue of reform itself could not be so easily avoided, but Gathorne Hardy was determined to approach it from an independent angle. He ordered his own investigation of the facilities for the sick poor in the city, and when the resulting reports recommended that a system of infirmaries and dispensaries be established, he dispatched John Lambert, a senior poor law inspector, to the one place in the United Kingdom where such a system was in operation – Ireland.

The idea that the Irish dispensary system might be relevant to English circumstances was not new in 1866. In the early 1850s several proposals that the Irish system be adopted in England were made both within and outside the House of Commons.[18] Subsequently a well-known medical reformer, Henry Wyldebore Rumsey, had repeatedly urged the establishment of a system of gratuitous medical relief for the bulk of the English poor.[19]

But the government, particularly the Poor Law Board, had never before been interested in such proposals. They had consistently defended traditional arrangements and denied that serious problems existed. Medical inspectors

[15] Ayers, *England's first state hospitals*, 7.
[16] Ibid. 8.
[17] Ibid. 10–11.
[18] *Hansard*, cxxix (1853), 134–6. See also Hodgkinson, *Origins*, 324–31.
[19] Ibid. 325–6.

were rejected as too expensive. The extension of free medical treatment to non-paupers was said to 'undermine motives for economy and forethought in the humble classes . . . and to slacken efforts for the preservation of that independence which is so essential to the respectability and true happiness of each individual'.[20] Some argued it would lead to the collapse of the private medical charities as well. Such arguments had served the board well for almost fifteen years, but attitudes toward poor relief were changing and in the mid-sixties they no longer appeared so automatically irrefutable. In that spirit Lambert was dispatched to Ireland in October 1866 to investigate the dispensary system and determine if, indeed, it was applicable to English conditions.

Lambert visited dispensaries in Dublin, Cork, Limerick and Galway, talked to medical officers, guardians and patients, and conferred at length with Alfred Power and the other poor law commissioners. He was most impressed. His report to Gathorne Hardy stressed the following points: the Irish dispensary system ensured the sick poor a sufficient supply of all necessary medicines and appliances; it provided both the mobile and confined patients with quick and convenient medical relief; it afforded full facilities for the compulsory vaccination programme; and it provided an organisation 'always ready, and capable of expansion if necessary, to meet any outbreak of epidemic disease'. Lambert concluded that

> after giving my best consideration to the system of dispensary relief, I am of the opinion that it is admirably adapted to the exigencies of large and densely populated communities, and I do not hesitate, therefore, to recommend that it should form an element of any scheme for the improvement of Poor Law Administration in this metropolis.[21]

Upon his return Lambert drafted and Gathorne Hardy guided through parliament what became known as the Metropolitan Poor Act of 1867.[22] Although limited to the Greater London area, the new measure marked a fundamental turning point in English poor law administration because for the first time it separated medical relief from traditional poor relief. Under its provisions separate institutions were to be provided for the insane and for patients suffering from smallpox and various form of fever. A network of dispensaries was to be established around the city in order to increase the availability of medical services and, it was hoped, reduce the threat of contagion by providing early care. These facilities and services were to be financed by a Common Poor Fund collected from each union in the city. Such an arrangement spread costs evenly and kept the poorer unions in the East End from bearing the brunt of the poor rates. Management of these new facilities

---

[20] *Hansard*, cxxix (1853), 136.

[21] *Lambert report*, 578–83.

[22] Webb and Webb, *English poor law history*, II/i. 334; *DNB* xvi. 459. Ayers attributes the entire bill to Gathorne Hardy (*England's first state hospitals*, ch. ii) but the Webbs and the *DNB* claim Lambert played the major role in its design.

was placed in the hands of a Metropolitan Asylums Board. Gwendoline Ayers concludes that without 'disrupting the structure of London's poor law administration, Gathorne Hardy had instituted a central hospital system which would confer preventive benefits upon all constituent localities, and a Common Poor Fund which would equalise their relief burdens'.[23] Actual implementation took both time and money. But by the end of the 1870s twenty infirmaries containing 10,000 beds had been built in the Greater London area as well as forty-seven dispensaries.[24]

The passage of the Metropolitan Poor Act increased the attention paid to the Irish dispensary system. With poor law infirmaries and dispensaries being established in London, advocates of widespread free medical care dared hope for the creation of a national dispensary system.[25] In that spirit the *Lancet* paraded the virtues of the Irish system before its readers with increased frequency, and appeals for liberalising state medical relief were renewed in parliament.[26] In this context Joseph Rogers, president of the English Poor Law Medical Officers Association, made two trips to Ireland in 1868 and 1869 and inspected the medical charities, particularly the dispensaries, first hand.[27] Impressed, he inspired a parliamentary return in 1870 comparing mortality rates in the three kingdoms, England and Wales, Scotland and Ireland for the period 1864–8. The figures surprised many. Mortality in Ireland was reported to be 1 in 60 of the population while in England it was 1 in 43.[28] More impressive were the comparisons of death rates for what were then termed zymotic diseases, that is infectious diseases like smallpox, scarletina, diptheria etc. England's figures were 1 in 190 while those for Ireland were 1 in 308. Subsequently Rogers went on to argue that the Irish figures were superior primarily as a result of twenty years of free, non-pauperising, state-run medical care. He held up the Irish dispensary system as a model upon which reforms in England should be based.

In retrospect we can see that the advantage in mortality rates between

[23] Ayers, *England's first state hospitals*, 28.

[24] Ibid.

[25] The Poor Law Board received a deputation of distinguished persons, 43 in all, mostly MPs led by the archbishop of York, on 23 July 1868. The matter under discussion was the treatment of sick paupers in workhouse infirmaries. Repeated reference is made to the Irish dispensary system: PRO, MH 25/19.

[26] *Lancet*, 1869, i. 690–91, 715–17. See also Hodgkinson, *Origins*, 328.

[27] Joseph Rogers, *Reminiscences of a workhouse medical officer*, ed. Thorald Rogers, London 1889, 94–7.

[28] *Return of estimated population and gross number of deaths registered for all causes; and from zymotic diseases in England, Wales, Ireland and Scotland in each year 1864–8* (HC 1870, lvi), 665. These ratios are given as presented in the return. A more conventional way to render them is as deaths per 1,000 or 100,000 of the population. Converted they are as follows. In Ireland the rate of gross deaths in the five years 1864–8 works out to 16.6:1,000 while that for England and Wales is 22.8:1,000. The rates for zymotic diseases are 3.3:1,000 and 5.2:1,000 respectively.

England and Ireland in the sixties, which so excited Rogers and like-minded reformers, was somewhat illusory. Irish mortality statistics were superior to those in England but not to the extent the reformers supposed at the time. The Births and Deaths Registration (Ireland) Act of 1863 appeared to have equipped Ireland with annual statistics comparable to those generated in England and Wales but in fact until 1879 it did not. The problem lay in persistent under-reporting which derived from weaknesses in the procedures at local level for reporting deaths. Adoption of an improved death certificate for use by coroners in 1876 and certain key provisions of the Public Health Acts of 1878 and 1879 requiring every 'Burial Board and Cemetery Company' to notify registrars of the district from which each of their bodies came, ended the problem.[29] But for the fifteen years between the publication of the first modern Irish statistics in 1864 and the onset of these reforms it appears that Irish mortality rates were understated by about 10–15 per cent annually. However, this problem was apparently not appreciated in the late 1860s and early 1870s when medical reformers were intent on the expansion of state medical care and hoped for the creation of something like a Ministry of Health. Then the Irish statistical advantage was taken to be true and, moreover, taken to be a result of the Irish combination of generous medical relief and central direction of epidemic control. Thus a *Lancet* editorial of 1870 concluded that

> After making all deductions, however, for the inevitable results of increased aggregation of population, it is difficult not to believe that the great inferiority of England's vital status to that of Ireland must depend . . . on inferiority in the means of dealing effectively with disease, especially zymotic disease, among the poor. The Irish Poor-law dispensary system supplies an efficient machinery, not merely for treating individual cases of disease that arise, but also for the constant watching (by means of an inspectorial staff who are periodically supplied with particulars of the public health in various districts) of zymotic diseases, which are the principal element in the preventable mortality of modern countries. And it must be boldly affirmed that in such matters as the great diminution of fever, and the practical stamping out of small-pox, which have distinguished the last decade of Irish medical history, the excellent Poor-law medical officers of Ireland have borne a most effective part.[30]

Growing and persistent outside pressure for a more generous system of state medical relief stimulated debate within the central poor law authority itself. The internal records of the Poor Law Board fail to reveal the full dimensions of the crisis but certainly suggest considerable disagreement over the direction state medicine should take. The question was whether something like the Irish dispensary system, that is non-pauperising state medical care through dispensaries separate from the workhouses, should be extended

---

[29] *Sixteenth annual report of the registrar general of Ireland, 1879* (HC 1880, xvi), 443–57.
[30] *Lancet*, 1870, i. 591–92.

throughout England and Wales. In 1868 Lambert's report on the Irish dispensaries was printed and circulated to all the English boards of guardians. In addition, the poor law inspectors were each instructed to give their views. By 1870 George Goschen, president of the Poor Law Board from 1868 to 1871, was led to wonder 'how far it may be advisable to extend gratuitous Medical Relief beyond the actual pauper class', and went on to suggest that

> The economical and social advantages of free medicine to the poorer classes generally, as distinguished from actual paupers, and perfect accessibility to medical advice at all times under thorough organisation, may be considered as so important in themselves as to render it necessary to weigh with the greatest care all the reasons which may be adduced in their favour.[31]

But this tentative move in the direction of a national health service failed to generate sufficient support, either within or outside the poor law administration, to push it towards completion. Neither the precedent of the Metropolitan Poor Act nor John Lambert's conversion nor Goschen's apparent interest was sufficient to achieve implementation of the Irish model on a national scale.

The opposition to comprehensive health care manifested itself at many governmental levels and was based on familiar objections. Leading the list was the view that free medical relief, generously applied, would undermine the independence of the working classes. In addition, critics claimed it would be ruinously expensive, would destroy the existing medical charities and self-help clubs, and was not even necessary in England anyway, given the availability of private medical care priced to accommodate all but the actually impoverished. Such attitudes were particularly characteristic of the guardians. Not until the end of the century was significant progress made in establishing separate poor law infirmaries and dispensaries outside the metropolis.[32]

In addition, resistance to any expansion of medical relief was strong within the poor law inspectorate in this period. John Lambert's enthusiasm for the comparatively generous Irish system appears remarkably modern when compared with the attitudes of the men with whom he worked. When asked whether the board should expand medical relief along the lines of the Irish system the inspectorate made its views clear. Inspector Hawley felt that the cost of medical relief for the sick poor was an item of 'serious and increasing amount in the Union accounts', and that if the medical officers were to achieve their goal of general relief expenditures would become 'utterly intolerable' and would so 'thoroughly disgust the ratepaying public as in the end to endanger or subvert the whole Poor Law Polity'.[33] His colleague,

---

[31] Webb and Webb, *English poor law history*, II/i. 322.

[32] Ibid. 320–1.

[33] Inspector Hawley to the Poor Law Board, 18 Aug. 1871, PRO, MH 32/43.

R. B. Cane, held roughly similar views arguing that expanding the freedom of the medical officers transferred 'a large proportion of Out-door relief from responsible to irresponsible hands . . . and effect a minimum benefit at a maximum expenditure'.[34] The reports of other inspectors echo these views though not all are as intransigent. Only W. A. Peel and H. B. Farnell were, in varying degrees, in favour of increased medical relief and the dispensary idea.[35] Thus Lambert's support of expanded medical care encountered stiff opposition within his own camp. In addition there were other arguments against dispensary medical relief. Among these was the growing resistance to increasing any form of outdoor relief.

In spite of the highly visible emphasis upon indoor relief championed by the central authority ever since the Royal Poor Law Commission's report in 1833, outdoor relief had continued to be a feature of English poor law practice at the local level where the guardians could, within reason, do as they wished. By the 1860s the increase in both private and public forms of outdoor relief had begun to alarm many both within and outside the poor law authority. However, by the end of the decade concern over too generous a policy had stimulated a fruitful co-operation between public and private charitable agencies which promised to reduce the need for conventional outdoor relief. By the arrangements worked out between the poor law authority and the Charitable Organisation Society, the latter would handle the needs of the worthy poor and the former would then tend to those that were left, that is to say, the chronically unemployable, through the workhouse test. It took some time for the details of this plan to be implemented, but by the late 1860s it was taking shape and promised to end the need for the usual forms of outdoor relief.[36]

In this context there was a clear attempt to tighten the administration of outdoor medical relief as well. The storm of criticism which had blown up over the management of the workhouse infirmaries in London in 1866 had led to the Metropolitan Poor Act and the repudiation of the idea of less eligibility for the sick. Hence poor law medical relief, both in the new, efficient and well-equipped and staffed 'state hospitals' constructed in London and in the refurbished workhouse infirmaries all over the country, became far more effective and generous in the 1870s than it had ever been before.[37] The improved quality of institutional relief mitigated against expanding outdoor relief in the minds of many. As the poor law inspectorate acclimatised itself to the increased emphasis upon quality medical care for

---

34 R. B. Cane to G. J. Goschen, president of the Poor Law Board, 24 Nov. 1870, ibid. 32/9.
35 W. A. Peel to G. J. Goschen, 20 Dec. 1870, ibid. 32/104; H. B. Farnell to G. J. Goschen, n.d. ibid. 32/24.
36 M. E. Rose, 'Crisis of poor relief', 61–2
37 Webb and Webb, x. 207–8.

the poor which became Poor Law and, later, Local Government Board policy from 1870 onwards, they were especially converted to the view that outdoor medical relief was now clearly inferior to the indoor care which could be provided more abundantly than in the past.[38] In this climate the other aspect of the Irish dispensary system, that is, non-pauperising medical relief, was clearly out of the question. Even persons associated with what we would now consider advanced ideas on most aspects of state medicine opposed such a policy. Thus the biographer of Sir John Simon, the pioneering medical officer to the Privy Council and later to the Local Government Board, observes,

> Simon never departed from the cardinal principle of less-eligibility even in health affairs. Whilst many other social reformers wanted the Poor Law medical service to become non-pauperising, he resolutely opposed this on principle and even in practice during minor local emergencies. In this respect, he clung to basic Poor Law doctrine, however socially irrelevant.[39]

Nevertheless, the idea that widely available medical care for the poor was sound social policy, the basic lesson of the Irish experiment, gradually gained support in England too. In spite of opposition from guardians, inspectors and even John Simon, non-pauperising medical relief haltingly but surely emerged as a feature of English poor law practice. Some support for it clearly existed at the Poor Law Board from the late sixties, and in the following decades circumstances progressively favoured its implementation. The official policy of the central authority remained hostile, but in practice substantial concessions were permitted.

For example, the London poor law hospitals, founded under the Metropolitan Poor Act of 1867 and originally restricted to paupers, were gradually transformed into general hospitals admitting anyone suffering from smallpox or other fevers. This policy was justified on the grounds that hospitalisation reduced contagion and hence served the public interest.[40] A royal commission supported the policy in 1881 and ten years later it was confirmed by statute, the Public Health (London) Act of 1891 (54 & 55 Vic., c. 76).[41] Even before this the government had removed an important penalty heretofore incurred by the poor when it determined that use of poor law medical services no longer disqualified a man from voting. Less progress was made outside the metropolis, but in 1879 the Local Government Board did grant rural boards of guardians the authority to admit non-paupers to poor law buildings if the facilities were technically transferred from the guardians acting as poor law authorities to the same individuals as public health

---

[38] Ibid.
[39] Lambert, *Simon*, 614.
[40] Ayers, *England's first state hospitals*, 82–5.
[41] Ibid. 92–3.

authorities.[42] In the latter capacity, which rural guardians were permitted to assume under the Public Health Act of 1875, patients could be treated without being pauperised. Hence, although a comprehensive network of poor law dispensaries was never established in England in the seventies and eighties, the poor law medical services gradually adopted practices consistent with the Irish approach through improvement in facilities and treatment as well as in broadening the right of participation. Much of this was a natural development of a tendency toward more generous state aid to the poor indigenous to English social and political thought at this time. Clearly, the Irish dispensary system did not act as a formal model towards which English reformers were shaping policy. However, as part of a package of ideas and evidence, it surely played a part in the evolution of poor law policy in these decades.

The extension of the Irish dispensary system to Greater London and the gradual liberalising of poor law medical relief in the 1870s were not the only aspects of the Irish system which influenced English attitudes in this period. In important ways it also affected the form taken by the next great restructuring of England's poor law and public health institutions, that is the creation of the English Local Government Board in 1871.

Of course Ireland had nothing to offer England regarding the core issues of Victorian public health policy – the establishment of clean water and air, garbage removal, and the other components of modern urban sanitation arrangements. The English had pioneered all this and Irish efforts in the nineteenth century were completely, and often inadequately, derivative. However, in other respects it appeared that the Irish Poor Law Commission's record in the 1850s and 1860s offered some useful ideas. Of particular interest was its success as the agency for epidemic control and vaccination which appeared to underline the advantages of centralisation at a time when the English were beginning to weigh the costs of decentralisation. The story of the development of public health reform in Great Britain is well-known and does not have to be retold here.[43] Yet a brief discussion of certain relevant details is essential in order to establish the context within which advocates of the Irish forms saw them working.

In the opening phase of the public health movement England had experimented with vesting broad powers in a central authority, the General Board of Health. Established by the Public Health Act of 1848, the general board

---

42 Webb and Webb, English poor law history, II/i. 325n.
43 The most recent comprehensive account is Wohl, Endangered lives. Other standard treatments are Simon, English sanitary institutions; Henriques, Before the welfare state; Frazer, English public health; and F. B. Smith, The people's health, 1830–1910, London 1979. Studies of key public health pioneers include: Brundage, England's 'Prussian minister'; John Eyler, Victorian social medicine: the ideas and methods of William Farr, Baltimore 1979; Finer, Chadwick; Lambert, Simon; and Richard A. Lewis, Edwin Chadwick and the public health movement, 1832–1854, London 1952.

was concerned with all aspects of public health from sewerage removal, piped water and garbage collection to epidemic control. Its efforts met with mixed success. On the one hand it did begin the long, difficult and costly process of facilitating the creation of modern systems of water supply and sewerage disposal despite the persistent resistance of local interests and authorities which objected to both the high cost and the imposition of what they perceived as a pushy central government.[44] Chadwick's authoritarian temperament and impatience with those who failed to respond to his vision made this approach difficult to bear yet slowly but surely by the mid-sixties the English population was being provided with improved water, air and general health services.

However, the General Board of Health did little to improve the nation's capacity to meet epidemics. It could issue orders under the Nuisances Removal and Diseases Prevention Act and its successors, but lacked the personnel and facilities to carry them out itself or the authority to force local agencies to do so. It was particularly in this area that England was so far inferior to Ireland. As we have seen the Irish Poor Law Commission coped admirably with the cholera in both 1853–4 and 1866–7. But the absence of a centrally controlled apparatus meant that the English response was far less satisfactory. Chadwick's frustration with the weakness of his board illustrates this point so vividly that it deserves extensive quotation. A report of the General Board of Health of 17 April 1854 on the recent cholera epidemic observed that while many local authorities had eagerly carried out whatever methods had been advised to prevent contagion, others had been blind and obstreperous:

> Instead of preparing to meet the danger, they shut their eyes against it. Cases of Diarrhoea occurring in unusual intensity, in unusual numbers, and at an unusual season, they regard as of no real significance. Successive deaths with the symptoms of malignant Cholera they call deaths from English Cholera as if changing the name altered the evil. They suppress, as far and as long as possible, the knowledge of all local forewarnings, whence a false security is maintained, which on the outbreak of pestilence, gives way to panic.

When one of the board's medical inspectors arrived in a district like this, he found the poor law medical officers overwhelmed. So occupied with the treatment of cases were they that

> they are wholly unable to devise, organise and superintend measures for preventing the spread of the pestilence among the population as yet unattacked. Additional medical assistance has now to be sought for at a distance, . . . house to house visitors to perform the service of bringing the premonitory cases under immediate treatment are to be obtained, houses of refuge are to be

---

[44] Wohl cites the case of Leicester where the local rates increased from 8d. in the pound in 1845 to 7s. in the pound between 1871–5: *Endangered lives*, 173.

obtained, dispensaries are to be opened; in short the whole preventive system has to be organised and before these arrangements can be made, which ought to have been completed before a single case of the disease occurred, the pestilence is at its height.[45]

Working from an inadequate and inaccurate theory of disease, lacking statutory power and personnel, faced with a population deeply resistant to central direction and control, the General Board of Health made many enemies. In 1854 Chadwick and his two colleagues were dismissed and four years later the board itself was broken up. The most important fragments were the Local Government Act Office, which was made administratively subordinate to the Home Office, and the Medical Department which was placed in the Privy Council. The former consisted largely of the sanitary branch of what had been the General Board of Health and the latter the medical branch. From 1858 until the formation of the Local Government Board in 1871, although statutes concerning sanitation, sewage utilisation, nuisances removal and disease prevention proliferated at a great rate, there was no single agency of the English government responsible for their implementation, supervision or coordination. Nevertheless, though the tone and emphasis of public health reform was significantly different from that of the Chadwick era, very important advances were made in those years. The reason lay largely in the achievements of Sir John Simon, medical officer to the Privy Council.

Simon (1816–1904) was a prominent pathologist who had begun his public career in 1848 when appointed first medical officer of health to the City of London.[46] Thereafter, he was made medical officer to the General Board of Health in 1855 and, with the dissolution of that body in 1858, moved to the Privy Council. Although Simon was as committed to reform as Chadwick and the other sanitarians, his ideas and approach were fundamentally different. As a medical man he was naturally sensitive to the scientific and medical aspects of public health problems for which Chadwick, the lawyer, had only contempt. While both men concentrated on the question of prevention, Chadwick had thought exclusively in terms of a common sense engineering approach, whereas Simon pioneered the modern concept of state medicine. Illustrative of the differences between them were their respective uses of mortality statistics. Chadwick considered disease purely a matter of the interaction of potent miasma with individual predisposition to a certain kind of illness. Remove the miasma and the problem was effectively solved. Chadwick had no further interest in the differences between various diseases. Crude death rates were therefore all he needed to know. The scientific–medical approach was very different. William Farr (1807–83), the brilliant statistician at the General Register Office from 1839 until 1880, pioneered

---

45 Quoted in *Third annual report*, 212.
46 Lambert, *Simon*, 99–111.

increasingly sophisticated methods of using mortality statistics to chart the nature of disease and the course of epidemics. Concentration upon the incidence and spread of specific diseases had produced important results by the 1860s. It was just such kinds of analysis which determined the water-borne nature of cholera in 1866.[47] Simon followed Farr in this kind of work. He and his staff constructed elaborate statistical breakdowns which revealed that factors such as contagion, occupation and overcrowding were vitally important to the incidence and spread of disease. Such discoveries suggested that sanitation was not the only solution to the problems of public health.[48] In the course of the sixties Simon extended his investigations to specific diseases such as diphtheria, tuberculosis, and small-pox. His scientific/statistical analyses probed the origins, dissemination and effects of these diseases upon the English population with unprecedented precision and thoroughness.

Moreover, Simon's revelations about the complexity and dimensions of England's health problems did not go unnoticed. His technical brilliance impressed politicians and public alike and in a fashion that the sanitarians' more commonplace and readily understood approach had not. The medical officer used this advantage to the utmost. He had an extraordinary ability to express his point of view both verbally and in writing. In his annual reports he used this skill to impress his readers with the need for further legislation. Gradually Simon's use of the emerging mystique of science succeeded in winning public approval for sanitary innovation where Chadwick's shrill demands for instant and massive change had failed.

One final factor which undoubtedly contributed to Simon's popularity and effectiveness was that he was, for most of his public career, not a centralist.[49] From the time he served as medical officer of health to the City of London, Simon had stood for local initiative in sanitary reform as against Chadwick's strong centralising programme. But even when operating within the structure of the national government at both the General Board of Health and the Privy Council his perspective remained much the same. Simon conceived the function of the central authority to be investigative. Once the facts about the incidence and propagation of disease were known, public opinion would produce appropriate legislative action at either the local or national level, whichever seemed the more useful and necessary. His own role was to provide the facts and interpret them to public and parliament alike. Simon eventually changed his mind about this, but the fact that he had been against centralisation for so long meant he did not incur the wrath of the anti-centralist clique which had brought down his belligerent predecessor.[50]

In the course of the late 1850s and early 1860s the public health move-

---

[47] Eyler, *Victorian social medicine*, 118–22.
[48] Lambert, *Simon*, 262–3.
[49] Ibid. 237, 241, 264–5.
[50] Ibid. 110, 207.

ment advanced in England but in a largely decentralised and unco-ordinated fashion. Local improvement, sanitation, water supply and sewage disposal measures were enacted at the request of specific towns and cities. Their importance in bringing an ever larger proportion of the population within the range of some sanitary authority was cumulatively impressive. Even on the national level some useful legislation took effect. The Local Government Act of 1858 gave local boards of health greater powers to hire medical officers and inspectors and to take preventive action. The Sewage Utilisation Act of 1865 created a whole new group of sewer authorities which not only affected rural areas for the first time but applied to Scotland and Ireland as well. A series of nuisance removal and disease prevention acts enlarged the powers of local authorities to deal with specific sanitation problems.

However, in spite of the obvious benefits of such legislation, the very proliferation of public health authorities, in the absence of overall direction from a central agency, created serious problems. Most of what sanitary reformers had wanted by way of legal powers was in existence by the mid-sixties, but enforcement was obstructed by the confusion resulting from the existence of so many overlapping agencies. Simon, despite his long-held convictions on local initiative, came to see the need for central direction. He described the complex of sanitary laws and jurisdictions as 'a parquetry which was unsafe to walk upon'.[51] And he ridiculed the absurdity of a code in which 'in each parish, the privies were under one authority and the pigsties under another'.[52] The immediate product of the medical officer's sense of the need for greater central direction was the Sanitary Act of 1866. That measure rendered compulsory much that had been optional and Simon, in a famous phrase, felt that English sanitary law had at last 'acquired the novel virtue of an imperative mood'.[53] The act was poorly drafted and did not work as well as was intended. However, in the late sixties this was of little moment. The attitude of the country with regard to public health reform was changing in much the same way as it was toward poor law medical relief. The public were prepared for fresh initiatives and new measures concerning the health of the nation across the entire spectrum of public policy.

In this context much was accomplished. A royal sanitary commission met in 1869. It made a number of recommendations which led in 1871 to the consolidation of poor law and public health agencies under one body, the Local Government Board, and to the further tightening and strengthening of sanitary law in the Public Health Acts of 1872 and 1875. Subsequently, similar statutes included Scotland and Ireland in the reorganisation and codification so that the entire United Kingdom came to operate under the same basic arrangements for public health law and administration. So sweep-

---

51 Simon, *Sanitary institutions*, 323.
52 Ibid. 321n.
53 Quoted in Fraser, *English public health*, 110.

ing and complete were the changes that they defined public policy in this area for a generation.

This was a creative and controversial period, the results of which did not satisfy everyone then or later. First and foremost among the critics was John Simon himself who, in his *English sanitary institutions* which first appeared in 1890, argued that the reforms were a betrayal of the recommendations of the sanitary commission and sold out medical to poor law interests. Subsequently, medical historians writing in this field have tended to follow Simon's lead. Both the reforms and the debate over them are relevant here because, as with the case of poor law medical relief, the Irish example appears to have played an important role in shaping the English government's response to the evident need for change. And, as with medical relief, the key individual was John Lambert.

John Lambert (1815–92) was far more important than his official position as a mere poor law inspector might suggest.[54] A solicitor, he joined the poor law authority as an inspector in 1856 and rapidly established himself as its most able career official. In 1864 he was relieved of conventional inspectorial duties, made inspector of audits, and assigned to the central office where his work was such, as he later wrote, as 'would generally be done by a Secretary'.[55] A gifted statistician, in 1865 he was called upon by Lord Russell, then prime minister, to calculate the electoral consequences of Russell's contemplated reform bill. Lambert supplied him with the figures. That measure died aborning but it launched Lambert on something like a second career as a confidential advisor to prime ministers on various pieces of legislation they had a mind. He served in this capacity for Gladstone and Disraeli when each in turn attempted parliamentary reform in 1866 and 1867. Subsequently, Lambert did the legwork for Gladstone's Irish Church and land acts of 1868 and 1870 respectively, worked with George Goschen, president of the Poor Law Board, on the Metropolitan Valuation Act, served on the Parliamentary Boundary Commission in 1868 and the Royal Sanitary Commission 1869–70, and on many other important commissions in the course of the 1870s and 1880s. By the late sixties he had achieved a reputation and influence far beyond the confines of the Poor Law Board. Gladstone, for whom he had done most of this kind of work, rewarded him in 1871 with the top permanent post in the new Local Government Board. He eventually accumulated the usual honours for outstanding service; he was made a CB in 1870 and a KCB in 1879.

Lambert's enthusiasm for the Irish medical relief system was based on many years work in the field of public health. As a member of Salisbury city

---

[54] There has been no biography of Lambert and he left no papers. The best treatments of his life and career are in Royston Lambert, *Simon*, 524–6, 536–9; Roy MacLeod, *Treasury control and social administration: a study of establishment growth at the Local Government Board, 1871–1905*, London 1968, 11–14; and Brand, *Doctors and the state*, 24–5.

[55] John Lambert, pension file, Treasury papers, PRO, T. 1/14398/7895/1883.

council in the early 1850s, Lambert led the fight to adopt the 1848 Public Health Act in the city. Then a young solicitor, he courageously took on the usual 'interests' who saw the act as a threat to their property rights and pocketbooks. The files of the General Board of Health reveal Lambert's tenacity in overcoming the council's resistance to the new measure.[56] His victory brought him public recognition and gratitude. On the occasion of his re-election the local paper congratulated 'Mr. Lambert, who has distinguished himself as the able, consistent, and unwearying friend of Sanitary Reform, and who has done so much to promote the drainage of the City.'[57] In recognition of his achievement the council elected Lambert mayor of Salisbury, an exceptional honour for a thirty-eight-year-old solicitor. But in addition it should be noted that Lambert was a Roman Catholic and that when he took the oath of office he became the first Catholic mayor of an Anglican diocesan city since the sixteenth century.

At the Poor Law Board Lambert was the source of some imaginative and progressive legislation. Sent to report on conditions in Lancashire during the cotton famine created by the Union blockade of Confederate ports during the American Civil War, he found them to be desperate. Mill operatives were faced with prolonged unemployment for which conventional poor relief was inadequate and inappropriate. Lambert recommended government subsidised programmes to employ labourers in public works. His reports formed the basis of the Union Relief Act (1862) and the Public Works (Manufacturing Districts) Act (1863) which provided the means to channel government funds to the workers.[58] Under the provisions of the latter act some £2,000,000 was channelled into the local economies in the hard-hit Midlands and employment found for more than 40,000 men. Equally if not more important, the money and labour were focused on sanitary works such as drains, sewers and pumping stations. Anthony Wohl argues that it was measures like this which stimulated local governments to take advantage of cheap loans which in turn accustomed them to moving forward on public health projects which might otherwise have been postponed.[59] These measures not only document Lam-

---

[56] John Lambert to the General Board of Health, 2 Feb. 1852, and John Lambert to J. J. Scott, clerk to the General Board of Health, 6 Apr. 1852, PRO, MH 13/160. See also T. W. Rammell, *Report to the General Board of Health on a preliminary inquiry into the sewerage, drainage, etc. . . . of Salisbury*, London 1851, 7–8, and the minute books of the Salisbury City Council 1847–53, Wiltshire Record Office.

[57] *The Salisbury and Winchester Journal*, 5 Nov. 1853.

[58] Lambert's role in this episode has been missed by historians largely because his reports have been misplaced and are not in his file among the poor law inspectors records nor in the records of the central authority. However, clear reference to his responsibility is made in his pension file (Treasury papers, PRO, T. 1/14398/7895/1883), and in a memorandum to the Treasury on the occasion of his appointment as permanent secretary to the Local Government Board (Hugh Owen to W. E. Baxter, Treasury secretary, 27 Nov. 1871, T. /7120B/18262).

[59] Wohl, *Endangered lives*, 174.

bert's sustained record as a sanitarian but illustrate his ability to adapt poor law machinery to novel and humane uses. His central role in the formulation and passage of the Metropolitan Poor Act is another such example.

Lambert's familiarity with the Irish dispensaries was reinforced in the late sixties by repeated trips to Ireland at the behest of Gladstone who was busy preparing his Irish Church and land measures. During 1868 and 1869 Lambert had occasion to visit all parts of the country. The experience only reinforced his initial impression of the Irish medical relief system. He wrote to Gladstone from Dublin in January 1869 that 'there is not much scope for improvement in the system of medical relief . . . and that I may add that the only good basis of organisation here is the Poor Law System'.[60]

In 1869–70 Lambert, in addition to his many other duties and activities, played an active role in the deliberations of the Royal Sanitary Commission, both serving upon it and testifying before it. The commission was the government's response to the growing demand for a rationalisation of public health policy and was charged both with investigating the nature of law and administration throughout the country at national and local levels, and with recommending appropriate measures for consolidation and improvement. To that end it met intermittently from April 1869 to June 1870, interviewed 101 witnesses, asked 12,436 questions, and submitted three reports totalling 1,456 pages of testimony, appendices and recommendations. It was the most important assessment of the nation's sanitary condition and health administration between Chadwick's 1842 report and the royal commission on the poor laws just before the First World War. And its recommendations led directly to the creation of the Local Government Board in 1871 and to the Public Health Acts of 1872 and 1875.

The Local Government Act of 1871 was merely organisational. It combined the Medical Department of the Privy Council, the Local Government Act Office, the General Register Office and the Poor Law Board into a single, comprehensive government agency – the Local Government Board – responsible for both poor relief and public health. The Public Health acts of 1872 and 1875 subsequently provided the new board with a comprehensive, simplified and enforceable sanitary code. Of the two the 1875 measure was by far the more significant. Earlier depicted as a pioneering statute, historians now see it as a consolidating act which rationalised and integrated the chaos of public health and sanitary legislation of the preceding two decades.[61]

Ireland was also affected by the effort to consolidate and reorganise poor law and public health institutions and laws. In 1872 an Irish Local Government Board was established and in 1874 and 1878 Irish Public Health acts were passed. The 1874 measure created stronger sanitary authorities in the

---

[60] John Lambert to William Gladstone, 29 Jan. 1869, Gladstone Papers, BL, Add. MS 44235.
[61] Fraser, British welfare state, 70.

towns and cities while that of 1878 consolidated existing Irish sanitary legislation and made the dispensary medical officers, medical officers of health in their respective districts.[62]

The fact that the Irish measures followed and in part were based upon those enacted in England has produced the impression among historians that Irish institutions and laws in this area were in general derived from English experience and initiative.[63] Insofar as sanitary matters were concerned England's influence is clear. Ireland produced no Chadwick or Simon, and all Irish sanitary legislation was ultimately based upon English precedents. But in other respects such a view is unsatisfactory, for in terms of the machinery for central supervision and control of a public health apparatus, Ireland had possessed a marked superiority over the English government since the passage of the Medical Charities Act in 1851. Consequently, the creation of the Irish Local Government Board required but superficial alterations to the character and functions of the Irish Poor Law Commission. A few titles were changed and some additions to its authority were made at the expense of the Irish Privy Council and lord lieutenant, but these were merely matters of detail and administrative streamlining. The Irish commission already possessed authority over birth and death registration, medical relief, public health and poor relief. In the words of the leading authority on Irish administration in the nineteenth century, 'In fact the new board was the poor law commission under a new name.'[64]

Such modest change was in marked contrast to that necessary in England, and the extent to which the new English Local Government Board of the seventies resembled the Irish Poor Law Commission of the previous decade is striking. Clearly the Royal Sanitary Commission had not intended that the English Local Government Board should be based explicitly on the organisational arrangement of the Irish Poor Law Commission. The commission saw its role as looking forward toward new and more effective ways of solving the problems at hand. Moreover, since much of the impetus for reform came from the medical community, the setting up of the Irish Poor Law Commission as a model would have been unlikely to generate enthusiastic support. State medical reformers like Rumsey may have admired the focus upon medical poor relief characteristic of the Irish dispensary system, but they were hostile to and suspicious of the poor law philosophy and the restrictive effect it was presumed to exercise on all forms of state medicine.[65] The medical interest therefore quite naturally pushed for a ministry of health more or less independent of poor law influence. None the less what they got was a Local

---

62 Evidence relating to Ireland, *Royal Commission report*, appendices, vol. x, 113–14.
63 Brendan Hensey, *The health services of Ireland*, 2nd edn, Dublin 1972, 8.
64 McDowell, *Irish administration*, 188.
65 Testimony of Rumsey before the Sanitary Commission, *First report of the Royal Sanitary Commission* (HC 1868–9, xxxii), 231–44.

Government Board effectively dominated by the senior administrators of its poor law component. That this was the case seems to have owed a great deal to the influence of John Lambert.

The Royal Sanitary Commission shied away from recommending a health ministry, which would have suggested a return to something on the lines of the still discredited General Board of Health. However, the commission did appear to recommend the creation of a new central authority divided into separate and equal departments for poor relief and state medicine. That would presumably mean that each department would have its own sphere of responsibility, staff and permanent officials each with equal access to the minister. Moreover, the medical community quite logically assumed that John Simon would be the senior officer in the medical department.

This was not to be the case however. Gladstone chose to intervene in the formative stages of the creation of the Local Government Board and the effect was to create a single secretariat with his protege Lambert at its head. The prime minister had been looking for an appropriate post with which to reward Lambert for some time. He thought so highly of him that he had put him up for the permanent secretaryship in the Treasury only to see Ralph Lingen get it instead. In 1882, on the occasion of Lambert's retirement from the board, Gladstone, then premier again, was consulted about the appointment of a successor. He claimed that the post was not in the gift of the crown and, therefore, not part of the patronage of the prime minister. The Local Government Board was given authority to make its own choice. Informed of this opinion by the then president of the board, J. G. Dodson, Lambert replied:

> Upon fuller consideration I am inclined to think that there was a special reason why the P. M. wished that when the LGB was established my appointment should come through him. I had been brought much in contact with him and done a great deal of work for the Gov't. and it had been a question whether I should not be appointed Sec. to the Treasury. If I am right this would account for the exceptional exercise of patronage by the P. M. on the first appointment of Sec. to the Board and make it clear, as I hope it is, that the present appointment rest with you.[66]

When the matter of constituting the new board came up in August 1871, Lambert's position was therefore 'extraordinary'. There was no question of dividing the secretariat in two and diluting his authority and role. However, in this process John Simon, though appointed medical officer to the board, found himself in a position of official subordination rather than equality. He was sufficiently cut off from what he took to be his traditional role as policy-

---

[66] John Lambert to J. G. Dodson, 25 Nov. 1882, Monk Bretton papers, Oxford, Bodl. Lib., Local Government Board III, box 52. See also E. W. Hamilton to J. G. Dodson, 7 Nov. 1882, ibid.

maker that he resigned in 1876. By the mid-seventies Lambert was the unchallenged ruler of all personnel below the president.

In this curious fashion England found herself equipped with an institution fundamentally similar to that which had long existed in Ireland. The Local Government Act had brought poor relief, medical relief and public health under one agency, as had the Medical Charities Act twenty years earlier in Ireland, and through the combined efforts of Gladstone and Lambert, the latter emerged with powers within the board very much like those of Alfred Power. The resignation of John Simon only reinforced the resemblance, for it robbed the agency of the one creative personality who might have led it in a different direction. With Simon gone his position was downgraded to a clearly advisory one, at a much reduced salary. Generally speaking, it came to resemble that of the medical commissioner on the Irish Local Government Board.

The establishment of the Local Government Board and the conflict between Lambert and Simon is a famous episode which has received a lot of attention from historians, none of it favourable to Lambert. It is relevant here because the anti-Lambert approach denies any creative or positive vision on Lambert's part; it insists on seeing Lambert in narrow, negative, traditional poor law terms, to which Simon's modern, scientific approach is sacrificed. The evidence bears another interpretation. It suggests that Lambert had a vision of public health administration which went well beyond traditional poor law policy and concerns and that this vision was constructive, moved English public health administration forward, was consistent with both the recommendations of the Royal Sanitary Commission and the political mentality of the time, and, finally, as with the matter of poor law medical relief, was influenced significantly by the record of the Irish Poor Law Commission in the area of public health in the previous two decades. This episode therefore needs to be examined in some detail.

First and foremost among the critics of the organisational arrangements and policy of the Local Government Board was John Simon himself. In his *English sanitary institutions*, Simon argued that the root of the problem lay in the way James Stansfeld, the first president, had constructed the new agency. Ignoring what Simon took to be the recommendations of the Sanitary Commission, Stansfeld chose to create a single secretariat responsible for both destitution and health, rather than separate and equal secretariats for each, and then compounded the error by permitting the old poor law officials to monopolise all the senior administrative posts. As Simon put it, 'it was as if the Act had ordered that the old Poor Law Board, subject only to such conditions of consultation and reference as itself might impose on itself, should be the Central Sanitary Authority for England.'[67]

According to Simon the effect of this arrangement was disastrous for the

[67] Simon, *Sanitary institutions*, 357.

public health interests of the nation. The poor law officials, he asserted, lacked a sense of urgency about health matters, were content with 'formal' rather than 'effective' action, and were insensitive to the need for expert medical opinion, something Simon saw as 'inherited' from their previous experience.[68] Writing fourteen years later Simon concluded 'I do not refrain from saying how grievously wrong I believe to have been the policy which that system represented . . ., I regard it as having been virtually a policy of retreat.'[69]

History has vindicated Simon. His conception of the role and importance of the medical officer has been validated by modern theories of disease and the methods appropriate to its control. And twentieth-century medical and administrative historians have seen his struggle in his own terms. Simon's biographer, Royston Lambert, reiterates and strengthens Simon's charges. The failures of the 1870s were 'due to the dominance of the Poor Law mind, to a shrivelling of attitude, a cooling of sanitary ardour . . . to a *contraction* in the exercise of unflinching state responsibility and in the confidence in state action'.[70] In one respect in particular modern historians go beyond Simon himself in assigning the blame for the suppression of state medicine: they place it not on Stansfeld but on John Lambert. Historians acknowledge Lambert's excellent adminstrative abilities but, none the less, insist on seeing him as an essentially poor law type. For example, Royston Lambert describes him as follows:

> Lambert lacked Simon's creative imagination and, as far as health and destitution matters went, had no long-term constructive ideals and asked no fundamental questions. He was much more interested in details, in organisation, efficiency and in perfecting machinery, than in the social purposes and needs which that machinery existed to serve.[71]

Jean Brand considers that it was Lambert's 'strong influence with Stansfeld [which] resulted in the Local Government Board's being organised on the stultifying outlines of the defunct Poor Law Board'.[72] And somewhat later she asserts that Local Government Board 'rigidity' was 'undoubtedly due to the authoritarian personality of John Lambert, a man who tended to regard all change as suspect'.[73]

This interpretation has had a long run. And, of course, it does reflect real aspects of the situation at the Local Government Board in the 1870s and in Lambert's personality and policies. However, it is, I contend, heavily skewed

---

[68] Ibid.
[69] Ibid. 392.
[70] Lambert, *Simon*, 541.
[71] Ibid. 525.
[72] Brand, *Doctors and the state*, 24–5.
[73] Ibid. 103.

in Simon's favour and has failed to acknowledge Lambert's very real record of achievement in the area of public health.

As we have seen, Lambert was not merely a poor law hack. Within the context of poor law officialdom he stood out as being exceptionally able and imaginative. George Goschen, the very competent and forceful president of the Poor Law Board between 1868 and 1871, and, thereafter, First Lord of the Admiralty, provides some hint at Lambert's importance in a letter to Gladstone on the occasion of his request, yet again, for Lambert's special services:

> In the dearth of men capable of doing real brain work I must cheerfully resign myself to losing Lambert's services for the time hoping that I may be able to retain them afterwards. But when in speaking of the abstraction of Lambert for a short time you say that you remembered that 'I have been, if I am not within an ace of losing him altogether', I hope you did not think that I should be able to carry on the business here minus Lambert without some man of ability being drafted into the department. . . . Pray do not think that I rely on Lambert to do any of *my* work and that *this is the reason* why I am so tenacious, but some support is necessary for the execution of one's plans and you know how badly off we are at the PLB.[74]

Subsequent heads of the Local Government Board like Stansfeld, George Sclater-Booth and J. G. Dodson echo these sentiments. Lambert was seen by the politicians he served as virtually irreplaceable. Even Robert Lowe, Gladstone's Chancellor of the Exchequer in 1871, and a strong supporter of Simon from their Privy Council days together, saw Lambert as the ideal man to carry out the wide-ranging duties that would be his on the new board and, indeed, specifically approved of uniting both health and destitution under his sole direction.[75]

There is no reason to think Lambert was prejudiced against the medical officer in particular or the Medical Department in general when he assumed his duties. He had, after all, been raised in a medical home for his father was a surgeon. But he had developed firm ideas about the role and place of the medical branch and they were very different from Simon's. Since this question was debated in detail in the protracted intra-office quarrel of 1873–6 we know quite precisely where each man stood. The correspondence between them and other interested parties runs to nearly fifty closely argued pages, most of it printed in the form of confidential memoranda. Boiled down it amounts to this.

---

[74] George Goschen to William Gladstone, 1 Dec. 1869, Gladstone papers, MS 44161, fo. 146.

[75] 'I think that it would give the experiment [the LGB] a much better chance of succeeding if the whole machine were placed under the signal ability of Lambert instead of bonding him with Fleming [another senior poor law official] who will give him no help and may encumber him': Robert Lowe to William Gladstone, 6 Sept. 1871, ibid. MS 44301.

Simon had had a position of virtual independence at the Privy Council for thirteen years and wanted the same freedom at the Local Government Board. He contended that the Royal Sanitary Commission had recommended separate and equal branches of health and destitution in the new agency and that, therefore, he should be given the authority to act as a permanent secretary and that the medical department should be administratively separate from the rest of the apparatus of the Local Government Board except that it would be responsible to the same minister. Lambert could run all the rest of the business of the board – poor law, poor law medical relief, local government, sanitary engineering, water and industrial pollution, etc. – as long as he left the medical department alone. In addition, Simon was unhappy with the way the board was conducting its sanitary programme. He argued that local sanitary authorities were lax about enforcing the law, that the board's general inspectors were incompetent in sanitary matters and should be replaced by medical inspectors under the medical department, that the board itself tolerated this general slackness and that the public health of the nation suffered as a consequence.[76]

On the other hand Lambert wanted a uniform and co-ordinated administration of all branches of the board under one hand. He argued that such an arrangement as Simon proposed was

> not only at variance with the principle of the Act of 1871, under which the several departments of Poor Law, Public Health, and Local Government have become amalgamated, but antagonistic to the scheme recommended by the Sanitary Commission . . . [which required that it was] . . . not only the health business that had to be kept together, but the entire business of the Board has to be administered as a consistent whole . . . [since] . . . the health business must necessarily be so mixed up with the general business of the Board that in many cases it would be almost impossible to define the limits with which each department would find itself called upon to act.[77]

Insofar as medical questions came within the work of the board they would be referred to the medical department for advice and inquiry 'just as engineering and legal matters would be referred to those respective departments for similar purposes'.[78] Lambert's case received strong and consistent support from the minister. When Stansfeld was replaced by George Sclater-Booth

---

[76] Simon's original memorandum to Stansfeld initiating the debate over office organisation does not survive. However, his position is presented in Stansfeld's memorandum of 23 June 1873, which summarises everyone's views and sides with Lambert, and in Simon's final appeal to Sclater-Booth of 10 Nov. 1875, which recapitulates his argument in great detail: PRO, MH 78/87.

[77] John Lambert to James Stansfeld, 10 Jan. 1873, Buchanan papers, reports on medical department staff, Department of Health and Social Services Library.

[78] Ibid.

upon the change in government in 1874, Simon started all over again and got precisely the same response. Why was this so?

Royston Lambert explains it in terms of John Lambert's forceful personality which, he claims, dominated both Stansfeld, described as 'weak', and Sclater-Booth who 'lacked force of character'.[79] This view slights both ministers and fails to assess the merits of Lambert's case, especially when viewed in the context of contemporary attitudes toward disease, medicine and the role of government.

Simon's claim that his proposals were within the spirit of the recommendations of the Sanitary Commission has been accepted from his day to our own. But when that document is examined closely there is surprisingly little evidence of such a commitment. The commission's report proper, as distinct from evidence of witnesses, appendices, tables etc., was issued in 1871. It consisted of four parts: (1) History of the sanitary laws; (2) Observations; (3) Suggestions for the new statute; and (4) Resolutions. Most of the passages relevant to the Simon–Lambert disagreement occur in the second and fourth parts. Simon's claim that the commission recommended a dual secretariat is based on two principal passages, Resolution 13, which states

> That it is expedient that the administration of the laws concerning the Public Health, and the Relief of the Poor should be presided over by one Minister as the Central Authority; whose title should clearly signify that he has charge of both Departments; an arrangement which would probably render necessary the appointment under him of permanent secretaries to represent the respective Departments.[80]

And, in the discussion of the nature of the new central authority, the assertion that though the subjects of public health and destitution are so necessarily intermixed in treatment 'that efficiency demands their final reference to one chief Minister, his title should clearly signify that his charge is of two distinct though correlative departments'.[81]

Those who have written on this question seem to have considered this suggested arrangement as binding and have further assumed that Simon would be that secretary. There is nothing in the report to indicate that the commission had such an idea in mind. On the other hand, we have Lambert's testimony, as a member of the commission, that such an arrangement was not contemplated.[82] And we have the evidence of Resolution 28 which states that the 'office of Chief Medical Officer under the Privy Council should be continued in the new department'.[83] In other words, that Simon should continue in the office and department he already occupied.

79 Lambert, *Simon*, 521, 548.
80 *Second report of the Royal Sanitary Commission* (HC 1871) xxxv. 175.
81 Ibid. 32.
82 John Lambert to James Stansfeld, 17 May 1873, PRO, MH 78/87.
83 *Second report of the Royal Sanitary Commission*, i, HC 1871, xxxv. 175.

But, more important, the report stressed the inter-relationship of poor law and public health matters. Finding that neither the Privy Council nor the Home Office were suitable places to house the central sanitary authority, the commission states that the 'Poor Law Board is in closest relation with every Parish in the kingdom upon matters intimately connected with the enforcement or neglect of sanitary measures.' Further that it has a staff of inspectors widely acquainted with the condition of every district, and a complete and efficient body of medical officers who could be made available where no other health officer is appointed for the purposes of Sanitary inquiry and information, and that the Boards of Guardians are the only available local authority in rural districts. These circumstances led them to conclude that 'the greater interests of efficiency demand an united superintendence and single responsibility for subjects so closely connected as the Public Health and the Relief of sickness and destitution among the Poor'.[84] In a memorandum on the role of the medical officers of health the commission concluded that 'our opinion coincides with that of the late President of the Poor Law Board, the Right Honorable the Earl of Devon, that "however the administration for the relief of the poor be improved, enlarged, or modified, there is no reason apparent why the sanitary functions might not usefully be added to that authority" '. It added 'It remains only to say under this head, that the existing arrangements of the Poor Law Board in Ireland . . . point to a similar conclusion.' [85]

Finally, the general tone of the commission's report needs to be taken into account. What strikes the modern reader is the general absence of references to state medicine as we understand it. This is a document overwhelmingly preoccupied with simplifying the law and with defining and organising local and central sanitary authorities. Scientific medicine was peripheral to the legal and administrative questions with which it was concerned. Medical men were involved, to be sure. The poor law medical officers were to be made medical officers of health and have much responsibility for local sanitary inspection, the new board was to have a medical department with a corps of inspectors, and medical men were thought to be useful in the role of experts and scientists whose special skills would be needed from time to time. The commission included five medical men, two of them, Henry Wentworth Acland and William Stokes, quite distinguished, so it cannot be accused of simply ignoring the medical dimension. But it is worth noting that the commission did not include Simon. And there is no evidence in its various reports and appendices that his conception of state medicine was in any way central to its thinking. Here again we need to ask why?

---

84 Ibid. 31.
85 Ibid. ii. 549.

By the early 1870s John Simon was the highly visible leader of the new wave of sanitary reformers – William Farr would be another – emphasising medical and scientific approaches to public health as distinct from the programme of clean water and new sewers pioneered by Chadwick and his supporters in the 1840s and 1850s. Yet while it is perfectly clear to us in the twentieth century that in the sixties and seventies Lister, Pasteur, Koch and others were assembling the evidence and developing the techniques that would demonstrate with crushing finality the validity of the germ theory of disease and the nature of sepsis, the question was far from settled in this decade. Simon and Farr were very sensitive to these new developments and early converts to germ theory, but many even in the medical profession were not. The pages of the medical journals are filled with the resistance of the unpersuaded. Let one example suffice. As late as 1876 the *Lancet* reviewed *Diseases of modern life* by Benjamin Ward Richardson, a distinguished physician and Fellow of the Royal Society. Described as a book which though intended for the public contains 'much to interest even the well-informed practitioner', the review goes on to report Richardson's conviction that ozone is the critical factor in much disease and that 'he looks forward to the time when by a careful comparison of the amount of ozone, [and] temperature, outbreaks of disease may be predicted at least as certainly as storms at sea'. 'The germ theory is dismissed as destitute of any foundation beyond a barren analogy.'[86] And so forth. By our standards Richardson was comically wrong about virtually everything. Yet in the year Simon resigned this work was taken seriously by the nation's leading medical journal.

In addition, Lambert was well aware of opposition to Simon among the other prominent sanitary reformers such as Edwin Chadwick and Florence Nightingale. Both considered Simon's ideas on disease 'superstition' and 'hypothesis and imagination' and in a letter to Stansfeld advised him to select men for the Local Government Board who had experience with 'real, practical sanitary work' and warned him against theoretical medicine, asserting 'that men with theories have absolutely no place in sanitary administration'.[87]

Perhaps even more important in undermining Simon's position at the Local Government Board was the 'expert' advice Stansfeld and Lambert received within the organisation itself. Edward Smith, a respected scientist who was also a Fellow of the Royal Society, and who since 1864 had been the medical officer to the old Poor Law Board, who knew Simon well, and had worked for him, wrote to Stansfeld in February 1873 objecting to Simon's whole way of proceeding.[88] According to Smith anything triggered an inves-

---

86 *Lancet*, 1876, i. 570.
87 Lambert, *Simon*, 522. See also Eyler, *Victorian social medicine*, 187–8. A useful discussion of the resistance of the English medical community to new ideas is contained in Youngson, *Scientific revolution*, chs v, vi.
88 The best treatment of Smith's life and work is T. C. Barker, D. J. Oddy and John

tigation, 'A letter from any person, official or otherwise, a report, a paragraph in the Newspaper a remark in the report of the Registrar-General . . . suffices to set them in motion.' He goes on to complain that Simon had reports issued under the heading ' "I am directed by the Local Government Board" but I have reason to believe that nearly all such inquiries are unknown at this institution. . . . Moreover, their nature is only such . . . as is fitting for the action of Local Inspectors of Nuisances'.[89] In the rest of a long letter Smith systematically attacks the very methods of immediate investigation of local outbreaks of disease by a highly trained medical expert with the authority of the central government behind him which lay at the heart of Simon's innovative approach and which, eventually, became a key component of successful public health procedure.

Though Smith's reputation was modest compared with Simon's, he was part of the same medical–scientific community. Divisions among the medical experts with respect both to the theory of disease and the role of the medical officers tended to discredit Simon's authority in the minds of laymen like Lambert and Stansfeld. Perhaps they would have agreed with the extreme sentiments of Alfred Power, Lambert's opposite number at the Irish Local Government Board and a seasoned veteran of sanitary administration. Writing to his old friend Chadwick about the terrible smallpox epidemic of 1872, Power complained of the ignorance of the Dublin hospital doctors who, he alleged, had broken up convalescent wards long before patients had ceased to be contagious and turned them out on the public. 'The mischief done both here and at Belfast by the Hospital Doctors in spreading the disease was incalculable.' And he goes on 'yet these are the fellows whom you, Rumsey, Acland, and Stokes (himself one of the Dublin culprits) would want to invest with a sanitary despotism, making them independent of the Local Boards of Management. The hardest whipping I have ever had to do has been to keep these boys in line.'[90]

Power may well have been wrong about the doctors' decision. At this distance in time there is no way of telling. But what is interesting about this quote is the attitude it reveals toward the professional judgement of distinguished medical men, in their own area of expertise, by a layman. Such a view would be unthinkable a generation later. But for men such as Lambert and Power, born in the first third of the nineteenth century, medicine and its practitioners commanded little respect when it came to understanding how to deal with epidemic disease. In the 1870s, as the germ theory of disease was in the process of being validated by the emerging science of microbiology, a

Yudkin, *The dietary surveys of Dr Edward Smith 1862–63: a new assessment*, London 1970. Also valuable is Carleton B. Chapman, 'Edward Smith (?1818–1874) physiologist, human ecologist, reformer', *Journal of the History of Medicine and Allied Sciences* xxii (1967), 1–26.
[89] Edward Smith to James Stansfeld, 18 Feb. 1873, PRO, MH 32/67.
[90] Alfred Power to Edwin Chadwick, 9 July 1872, Chadwick papers, University College Library, University of London.

seismic change was taking place in the theoretical underpinnings of the medical profession. But we have to forgive Lambert, Power and many others who did not appreciate the significance of the change.

In conclusion, I think we can broaden our understanding of this episode in particular, and sanitary reform in England in the 1860s and 1870s in general, if we step back from the good guy/bad guy approach which has characterised it thus far and recognise: (1) that Lambert was not necessarily an enemy to public health because he opposed Simon's claims to administrative equality and some of his ways of proceeding with the duties of his office; (2) that his administration of Local Government Board sanitary policy was consistent with the recommendations of the Sanitary Commission, in some respects more consistent than Simon's ideas; and (3) that until the medical community clearly agreed on the nature of disease, the conflicting approaches to state medicine advocated by different but equally distinguished members of the profession confused laymen and precluded decisive action. Thus in the 1870s government officials were left with what they could understand and what they took to be the recommendations of the Sanitary Commission – legal and administrative uniformity, central supervision and local enforcement. Though less scientific than Simon's approach it represented, none the less, a positive step forward, a constructive policy which achieved much in the following decades. In addition, it needs restating that Lambert's experience with the Irish Poor Law system in the late 1860s appears to have contributed to his view that the poor law administrative apparatus, local and central, was uniquely fitted to carry out the sanitary work of the country. Time quickly proved this to be a mistaken notion. The rapid growth of scientific medicine in the last two decades of the century vindicated Simon's assertion of the primacy of the medical expert and of the need for vigorous, centralised administration and enforcement of sanitary law. But Lambert and the other sanitarians of the 1870s must be understood in their own terms, not as narrow reactionaries and bureaucratic power brokers but as good men intent on improving the health of the nation by methods which they took at the time to give good results and which were politically more in the mainstream than those of their critics.

Conclusion

The zeal for centralisation which had gripped Irish medical charity reformers in the mid-1830s, gradually subsided in the 1870s in the wake of the creation of the Irish Local Government Board (1872). Clearly the changes that had been made since 1851 had much to do with the reduction in interest in further change. Many concluded that application of existing laws and institutions rather than further reforms was what was most needed. Yet there was also a loss of imagination and vision. Sir Alfred Power retired from the Irish Local Government Board in 1879, Sir John Lambert from his post three years later. Their successors were no doubt competent men but it is clear in retrospect that something vital went out of both organisations with the loss of these men. In particular the creative effort to improve the state's role in medical relief and epidemic control atrophied in the 1880s and 1890s. Innovation and experimentation were replaced by administration and routine. Why? A number of reasons suggest themselves. Christine Bellamy argues that the problems were largely structural.[1] Her recent study of the English Local Government Board from 1871 to 1919 stresses the extent to which its administrators were hampered by restrictive fiscal policies and what she calls the complex 'culture' of central–local relationships which, in spite of the strengthening of the legal powers of the central board by that period, none the less favoured the local authorities. My reading of the mentality of the board's leadership supports this view. The failure of the General Board of Health to gain the support of local authorities was a powerful living memory in the 1870s and conditioned the approach adopted from 1871 onward. The Sanitary Commission reports reveal the high degree of compromise with the local level. While consolidating the heretofore dispersed poor law, sanitation and state medical agencies into a single body which had the appearance of a powerful engine of state centralisation, the mentality of the senior officials was in fact what Bellamy labels 'diplomatic–political', an approach which stressed negotiation rather than confrontation with local officials.[2]

The generational shift may also have been important. Power and Lambert, like Chadwick and Nightingale, were products of the public health reform enthusiasm of the mid-century. They were, though in a more modest way, crusaders who were convinced that sanitary reform under the direction of

---

[1] Christine Bellamy, *Administering central–local relations, 1871–1919: the Local Government Board in its fiscal and cultural context*, Manchester 1988, 11–12.
[2] Ibid. 15.

central government could solve the public health dilemmas of their time. They fought both vested interests too narrow to understand the need for change and a medical profession which was divided over its various theories of disease propagation and treatment and resentful of lay intrusion and control. They were largely successful on both fronts by the 1870s. But their victory was mixed. If it had become clear by the 1880s that public health lay largely in cleaning up water and air, the environmentalist approach advocated by sanitationists from the beginning, then that very victory negated the need for more innovation and reform. Application of the existing sanitary laws would do the trick. Moreover, the centralising trend was exhausted. Public opinion now largely recognised that the expense of drains and piped water had to be borne, though less so in Ireland than in England, but would have the initiative vested in the local authorities responsible for raising the rates and contracting the works. Sound administration of existing law, not continued reform and agitation, was the perceived need of the day.

Finally, in complex ways the triumph of germ theory in the 1870s may have abetted the move toward passivity on the public health front. If, on the one hand, it showed that the sanitary idea was right insofar as it justified the public health measures already on the books, it also demonstrated that leading sanitarians like Chadwick had been fundamentally ignorant although the measures they had advocated had been correct. It showed that disease was not a matter merely of smells but of specific microscopic creatures, invisible yet pervasive. Coping with the challenges presented by such life forms was not work for lawyers but for scientists trained and equipped to identify and develop defensive measures against the most dangerous of them. Thus the emergence of germ theory turned victory into defeat for the sanitarians. Having wrested control of public health administration from the doctors they now had to acknowledge the primacy of medical science on the theoretical front. Had John Simon held on for another few years he might have captured the new wave and used it to gain the independence and control he had fought for between 1871 and 1876. But he was gone by 1876 and no one like him challenged the public health administrators in the 1880s and 1890s.

Public health historians must be forgiven for failing to detect any connection between the coming of the English Local Government Board in 1871 and the Medical Charities (Ireland) Act of twenty years earlier. The significance of the Irish Dispensary system for reforms in England has been misunderstood for a variety of reasons. In part the name itself is misleading suggesting merely a form of out-door medical relief. In fact, as we have seen, it was very much more than that combining poor law, medical care and public health services within a highly centralised agency. John Lambert appears to have understood it in these comprehensive terms, and he was the key player in the whole process: the most influential figure in the poor law authority, the best informed regarding the Irish system, a member of the Sanitary Commission, the principal architect of the new Local Government Board, and its dominant civil servant for the first decade of its existence. For him the Irish system appeared to offer the answer to most of the problems facing the English poor law authority and English sanitarians in the late 1860s. Even the doctors, or at least some of them, were impressed. Not only would it provide systematic, out-door medical relief but the consolidation of poor law and public health institutions and personnel under a central director, backed by statute, in turn promised improved epidemic control. Thus when the rapid changes which took place in English public health law are examined in the period between 1867 and 1880 it is the degree to which they conform to the Irish institutional structure of the mid-sixties which strikes the eye. The Metropolitan Poor Act (1867) provided for the creation of infirmaries, isolation hospitals and dispensaries, at least in London, and infirmaries in the important provincial towns; the gradual non-pauperisation of poor law medical relief, turning it into state medical relief; the consolidation of medical, public health, sanitation and poor law services under one agency controlled by poor law officials. Thus the English welfare administration came to acquire by 1871 the structure built up in Ireland in the previous twenty years. Naturally the fit was not exact. History is not neat nor does it seem necessary for the historian to require exact duplication in order to argue that we have here a good example of the kind of thing W. L. Burn had in mind when he argued in his 1948 article that Ireland served as a kind of laboratory for administrative forms later adopted in England.[3]

Historians have missed the Irish connection for a variety of reasons; partly because they have not been looking for it, partly because they had little reason to think Ireland more advanced in any sector of medical relief or public health in this period than England, and partly because there is little obvious evidence for it. With the exception of Lambert's 1867 report, and the works of Rogers and Rumsey, none of the works of the contemporary reformers involved pointed in Ireland's direction. For the most part public attention at the time, and that of historians later, was focused on the work of Simon and the Sanitary Commission.

A couple of other interpretative issues raised in the study deserve final comment. Though now rather out of fashion, it was the debate over the Victorian revolution in government which inspired and shaped the early stages of my research. Central to that revolution, though seldom stressed by historians, was the shift in thinking from local to national scale and from particular to general categories. The reform of the Irish medical charities illustrates this shift particularly well. The pre-1830 Irish medical charities were a considerable achievement. As MacDonagh and others have suggested, and as this study shows, the variety, number, distribution and funding of these institutions and the numbers of people they served was impressive testimony to the extent of private philanthropy and the initiative of both local and

---

[3] W. L. Burn, 'Free trade in land: an aspect of the Irish question', *Transactions of the Royal Historical Society*, 4th ser. xxxi (1949), 68.

national governments. Yet by the 1830s growing numbers of concerned and influential persons were persuaded that the medical charities were deeply flawed and required substantial reformation. By eighteenth-century standards there was little to complain about. But by the tests of the 1830s and 1840s, nearly everything appeared to need changing. What had happened? Clearly the standards against which the efficiency of the medical charities was measured had changed. They had been established by statute but had actually been brought into being as a result of local initiative and local money. Consequently, their distribution and the arrangements under which each of them functioned were unsystematic and varied. The critics of the 1830s medical charities found such local and regional variation anathema. They wished to substitute minimum standards in all important areas and categories of medical charity operation and administration. They thought in comprehensive and national terms. Why? One source is clear. Insofar as they were influenced by utilitarianism it led them to wish to establish uniform standards regarding geographical distribution, financial support for facilities, medicines, salaries and the qualifications of medical personnel. But even without self-conscious adherence to such ideas, the effect of systematic scrutiny of the medical charities across the length and breadth of Ireland led the investigators to concoct a scheme of national minimal standards within which they could frame their recommendations for reform. Thus the investigating team of the Whately Commission and the reforming apothecary, Denis Phelan, came to essentially the same conclusions and recommended roughly the same solutions. And when the new poor law was established in Ireland in 1838, the central authority saw the solution to the medical charities problem in the same terms and, naturally, saw itself as the agency to administer an improved national system. Who was motivated by what theory of government is impossible to determine. What is striking is the extent to which the very process of investigation necessarily led to conceptualisation in terms of a national system and to the framing of minimum standards for each of the important aspects of medical charity organisation, administration and operation. Once so framed the reform proposals came to define the parameters of the debate from then on, or at least until the creation of the Irish Local Government Board in 1872.[4]

Another theme which emerges in the course of examining the efforts to reform the medical charities, both before and after 1851, is the effect that process had upon the professionalisation of the Irish medical community. The aggressiveness with which the doctors defended what they took to be their turf is particularly striking. From the outset elements of the profession, particularly the Irish College of Surgeons, took the lead in articulating ad-

---

4 This view is compatible with, while not being quite the same as, that put forward by MacDonagh in his famous article. MacDonagh, 'The Nineteenth Century Revolution in Government: A Reappraisal', *Historical Journal*, I (1958), 52–67.

vanced positions *vis à vis* both the administration of the medical charities and the kind of service they should provide. This persistent battle, raging over several decades, had important implications for the ways in which the doc-tors thought about themselves and their profession as well as for their role in the administration of medical charity and in the nature of care they were to provide. On the one hand the effect of the wide-ranging investigations of the 1830s and 1840s was to convince the doctors that they faced the threat of subordination to some kind of central authority, most ominously from their perspective, that of the new poor law. That threat forced a more or less rapid reconsideration of priorities within the medical community resulting in the beginning of the process of mending of ancient divisions among the tradi-tional categories of practitioners as well as the articulation of advanced positions on both the quality and quantity of the relief medical officers should be permitted to provide. The founding of the *Dublin Medical Press* and the Irish Medical Association in 1839 and the creation of the first chair of public health in the United Kingdom by the Irish College of Surgeons in 1841 are particularly good examples of this process. On the other hand, as recent research has demonstrated, other factors were at work, pre-eminently the rise of the general practitioner and the agitation for medical reform. Yet the Irish case suggests that the emergence of the new poor law played a central role in driving the doctors toward a professional framework from within which they could advance their case most successfully.

In addition, the impact of the new poor law was intriguingly complex and contradictory. If it frightened the medical men and thus promoted internal fence-mending and co-operation, it also created medical facilities and jobs at a time when the supply of doctors easily outstripped demand. In the case of Ireland, for example, even before the passage of the Medical Charities Act, the central authority had dramatically increased the number of fever hospitals. Once in charge of the dispensaries it persistently extended medical service through increases in facilities and personnel even as the population declined in the 1850s and 1860s. And, failing in its bid to acquire the county infirmaries, the Poor Law Commission moved to convert the workhouse infirmaries into general hospitals treating paupers, the poor and paying customers alike.

In England too, as Michael Flinn has noted, though the new poor law made no provision for medical relief the 1830s in fact witnessed something like the founding of the poor law medical service as boards of guardians routinely appointed medical officers to serve the newly-formed unions.[5] Even more wretchedly funded in proportion to total expenditures than its Irish counterpart, nevertheless it achieved grudging recognition in the following decades. The General Medical Order of 1842 defined standard medical dis-tricts and recognised the area of medical relief as a poor law responsibility.

---

[5] M. F. Flinn, 'Medical services under the new poor law', in Derek Fraser (ed.), *The new poor law in the nineteenth century*, London 1976, 48–9.

Recognition brought instant expansion. Vaccination through the poor law medical service was introduced in 1840, made compulsory in 1853, and considerably toughened in 1867. The Nuisances Removal and Diseases Prevention Act of 1846 made rural guardians responsible for cleaning up their unions, tasks which inevitably fell largely upon the medical officers. The reforms of the late sixties, which established the metropolitan poor law infirmaries and dispensaries, strengthened the medical and public health functions of the poor law to the point where it becomes clear that medical care and public health duties emerge as a major responsibility of the state.

As a consequence of this process thousands of medical men found employment in the poor law medical services in both England and Ireland. Though doubtless welcoming the income, their conditions of employment were such as to perpetuate resentment and anxiety. Underpaid and often bullied by the guardians and the central authority, the doctors maintained a curiously paradoxical relationship with the poor law. The creation of the Poor Law Medical Officers Association in the 1860s provided them with an organisation through which they could press their grievances. Though tangential to the main focus of this study, this interestingly adversarial relationship invites further research. The evidence suggests that the pressure supplied by the poor law may have contributed substantially toward the definition of medical identities and interests. In addition, such research should not neglect to include regions outside of England. The history of the Irish medical charities and the poor law system which largely replaced them in 1851, illustrates the inter-relatedness of the poor law and the medical communities in the United Kingdom.

Bibliography

Unpublished primary sources

Cork, Cork County Archives
Records of the Board of Guardians, Cork Union

Dublin, National Library of Ireland
Larcom papers
Mayo papers
Monteagle papers

Dublin, Royal Irish Academy
Haliday pamphlet collection
Tracts

Dublin, State Paper Office
Chief secretary's office
Departmental letter books
Official papers
Registered papers
Chief crown solicitor's papers

London, British Library
Gladstone papers
Nightingale papers

London, Department of Health and Social Services Library
Buchanan papers

London, University College Library
Chadwick papers

Oxford, Bodleian Library
Acland papers
Clarendon papers
Disraeli papers
Monk Bretton papers

Public Record Office, Kew
Ministry of Health records
MH 13 General Board of Health and Local Government Board correspondence
MH 19 Correspondence and papers with other government offices, 1834–1908
MH 25 Miscellaneous correspondence and papers
MH 32 Correspondence of assistant poor law commissioners and inspectors
MH 78 Establishment and organisation, 1862–1924

Treasury Board papers
Trevelyan papers

Salisbury, Wiltshire Record Office
Minute books of the Salisbury City Council, 1847–53

Published primary sources

Annual reports
Annual reports of the Irish Poor Law Commissioners and Local Government Board, 1848–80
Annual reports of the Irish Poor Law Commissioners under the Medical Charities Act, 1853–9

Other parliamentary papers (in chronological order)
1805, vol. i, *Bill to amend an act for erecting infirmaries and hospitals in Ireland*
1813–14, vol. ii, *Bill for further encouragement of fever Hospitals in Ireland*
1818, vol. ii, *Bill for establishing and regulating fever hospitals in Ireland*
1818, vol. ii, *Bill to amend acts for establishing county infirmaries in Ireland*
1818, vol. vii, *Report from the select committee appointed to inquire into the state of Ireland as to the prevalence of contagious fever in that part of the United Kingdom, and to investigate the causes . . . and to secure adequate means of support to the establishments destined for the relief of the diseases*
1819, vol. viii, *Report of the committee appointed to take into consideration the act passed in the last session . . . for regulation of grand juries in Ireland*
1830, vol. vii, *Report of the select committee of the House of Commons on the state of the poor in Ireland*
1831–2, vol. xlv, *Return of the fever hospitals in Ireland for the reception of fever patients only, receiving public aid, either from parliamentary grant or local assessment*
1833, vol. ii, *Bill to explain and amend the provisions of certain acts for erecting and establishing public infirmaries, hospitals and dispensaries in Ireland*
1835, vol. xxxii, pt ii, *First report of the commissioners inquiring into the condition of the poor in Ireland, appendix (B): Public medical relief, dispen-*

saries, fever hospitals, lunatic asylums, etc.; with supplement, pts i, ii containing answers from officers of medical institutions

1836, vol. iv, Bill for the regulation of medical charities supported by county assessment

1837, vol. iii, Bill for the better regulation of hospitals, dispensaries and other medical charities in Ireland

1837, vol. xxxi, Second report of the commissioners for inquiring into the condition of the poorer classes in Ireland

1837–8, vol. iv, Bill for the better regulation of hospitals, dispensaries and other medical charities in Ireland

1840, vol. iii, Bill to extend the practice of vaccination in Ireland

1840, vol. iii, Bill to prevent inoculation for small pox and to extend the practice of vaccination

1840, vol. clviii, Abstract of returns of total annual income and expenditure of every fever hospital in Ireland, 1835 to 1837; showing number of patients, establishments, governors, etc

1840, vol. xlvii, Abstract of grand jury presentments

1841, vol. li, Report of the poor law commissioner on the medical charities (Ireland)

1842, vol. iii, Bill for the better regulation and support of the medical charities in Ireland

1843, vol. iii, Bill for the better regulation and support of the medical charities in Ireland

1843, vol. x, Report of the select committee of the House of Commons on the Irish medical charities

1846, vol. xi, pts i, ii, Report by the Lords' select committee appointed to inquire into the operation of the 1 & 2 Vict. c. 56, and the other laws relating to the relief of the destitute poor in Ireland; and also to inquire into the operation of the medical charities in Ireland

1849, vol. xv, Fifteenth report of the select committee of the House of Commons on the poor laws (Ireland)

1850, vol. iv, Bill for the better distribution, support and management of the medical charities in Ireland

1850, vol. li, Abstract of returns of the number of temporary fever hospitals still kept up in each union in Ireland under the Act 11 & 12 Vict. c. 131, . . . the number of fever hospitals supported by the poor rate; and the number of dispensaries, fever hospitals, and infirmaries, for which county presentments were made in 1849

1851, vol. iv, Bill for the better distribution, support and management of the medical charities in Ireland

1857–8, vol. iii, Bill to amend the laws in force for relief of the destitute poor in Ireland

1861, vol. x, Report of the select committee on poor relief (Ireland)

1862, vol. xlix, Reports from medical inspectors in 1861 and 1862 on the poor in Roscommon, Sligo, Galway and Mayo

1867, vol. lx, *Report on the system of medical relief to out-door poor under the Dispensaries Act of 1851*

1868–9, vol. xxxii, *First report of the Royal Sanitary Commission*

1871, vols i–iii, pt i, *Second report of the Royal Sanitary Commission*

1870, vol. lvi, *Return of estimated population and gross number of deaths registered for all causes; and from zymotic diseases in England, Wales, Ireland and Scotland in each year 1864–8*

1874, vol. iii, pt ii, *Second report of the Royal Sanitary Commission*

1878–9, vol. xxxi, *Report of the Poor Law Union and Lunacy Inquiry Commission (Ireland)*

1880, vol. xvi, *Sixteenth annual report of the registrar general of Ireland, 1879*

1910, vol. i, *Report of the Royal Commission on the poor Laws and relief of distress*, appendix ii, *Poor law dispensary medical relief in Ireland*

Newspapers and Periodicals

British Medical Journal

Dublin Medical Press, 1839–59; *Dublin Medical Press and Circular*, 1860–5; *Medical Press and Circular*, 1866–

Dublin Quarterly Journal of Medical Sciences

Freeman's Journal

Lancet

Local Government Board Chronicle

London Medical Gazette

Medical-Chirurgical Review

Salisbury and Winchester Journal

Contemporary books and articles

Acland, Sir Henry Wentworth, *National health*, Oxford 1871

———— *The public health*, Oxford 1880

Clarke, James F., *Autobiographical recollections of the medical profession*, London 1874

Harrison, Robert and Dominic J. Corrigan, *Observations on the draft of a bill for the regulation and support of medical charities in Ireland*, Dublin 1842

———— *Supplement to observations on the draft of a bill for the regulation and support of medical charities in Ireland*, Dublin 1842

Ingram, J. K., 'Comparison between the English and Irish poor laws with respect to conditions of relief', *Journal of the Statistical and Social Inquiry Society of Ireland* iv (1864), 43–61

Jacob, Archibald H., 'The poor law medical charity system of Ireland', *Dublin Journal of Medical Sciences* lxxxi (1886), 204–23

Medicus, *Observations and suggestions on the medical charities of Ireland*, Dublin 1851

Nicholls, Sir George, *A history of the Irish poor law*, London 1856, repr. 1967

Phelan, Denis, *A statistical inquiry into the present state of the medical charities of*

Ireland with suggestions for a medical poor law by which they may be rendered much more extensively efficient, Dublin 1835

———— *Reform of the poor law system in Ireland or facts and observations on the inadequacies of the existing system of poor relief*, Dublin 1859

Power, Alfred, *Sanitary rhymes, personal precautions against cholera, and all kinds of fever*, London 1871

———— *A paper on outdoor relief in Ireland, prepared at Earl Spencer's request*, London 1875

Rannell, T. W., *Report to the General Board of Health on a preliminary inquiry into the sewerage, drainage, etc., . . . of Salisbury*, London 1851

Rogers, Joseph, *Reminiscences of a workhouse medical doctor*, London 1889

Rumsey, Henry Wyldbore, *On state medicine in Great Britain and Ireland*, London 1867

Simon, Sir John, *English sanitary institutions*, 2nd edn, London 1897

Sprigge, S. S., *The life and times of Thomas Wakley*, London 1897

Stewart, Alexander and Edward Jenkins, *The medical and legal aspects of sanitary reform*, London 1867 (repr. with an introduction by M. W. Flinn, New York 1969)

Stokes, William, *William Stokes, his life and work, 1804–78*, London 1898

Thomson, William, 'The Irish poor-law medical service', *Dublin Journal of Medical Science* ci (1896), 193–202

Walpole, Sir Spencer, *Life of Lord John Russell*, 2 vols, London–New York 1891

Secondary sources

Abel-Smith, Brian, *The hospitals 1800–1948: a study in social administration in England and Wales*, Cambridge, Mass. 1964

Agnew, L. R. C., 'Scottish medical education', in C. D. O'Malley (ed.), *The history of medical education*, Berkeley–Los Angles 1970

Atlay, J. B., *Sir Henry Wentworth Acland, Bart, KCB, FRS, Regius Professor of Medicine in the university of Oxford: a memoir*, London 1903

Ayers, Gwendoline M., *England's first state hospitals and the Metropolitan Asylums Board 1867–1930*, Berkeley–Los Angeles 1971

Barker, T. C., D. J. Oddy and John Yudkin, *The dietary surveys of Dr Edward Smith 1862–63: a new assessment*, London 1970

Barrington, Ruth, *Health, medicine and politics in Ireland 1900–1970*, Dublin 1987

Beckett, J. C., *The making of modern Ireland 1603–1923*, London 1966

Bellamy, Christine, *Administering central–local relations, 1871–1919: the Local Government Board in its fiscal and cultural context*, New York 1988

Best, G. F. A., *Shaftesbury*, London 1964

Bishop, W. L., 'The evolution of the general practitioner in England', *The Practitioner* clviii (1952), 171–9

Black, R. D. Collison, *Economic thought and the Irish question*, Cambridge 1960

Blake, Robert, *The Conservative party from Peel to Churchill*, New York 1970

Blaug, Mark, 'The myth of the old poor law and the making of the new', *Journal of Economic History* xxiii (1963), 151–84

Brand, Jeanne L., *Doctors and the state: the British medical profession and government action in public health, 1870–1912*, Baltimore 1965

Brebner, J. B., 'Laissez-faire and state intervention in nineteenth-century Britain', *Journal of Economic History* viii (1948), 59–73

Briggs, Asa, 'The welfare state in historical perspective', *Archives Européennes de Sociologie* ii (1961), 221–58

Brooke, Charles W., *Battling surgeon*, Glasgow 1945

Bruce, Maurice, *The coming of the welfare state*, London 1961

Brundage, Anthony, *The making of the new poor law*, London 1978

––––––– *England's 'Prussian minister' Edwin Chadwick and the politics of government growth, 1832–1854*, London 1988

––––––– David Eastwood, and Peter Mandler, 'Debate: the making of the new poor law, *redivivus*', *Past and Present* cxxvii (1990), 183–201

Burn, W. L., 'Free trade in land: an aspect of the Irish question', *Transactions of the Royal Historical Society* 4th ser. xxxi (1949), 61–74

––––––– *The age of equipoise*, London 1964

Cameron, Sir Charles A., *A history of the Royal College of Surgeons in Ireland and of the Irish Schools of Medicine*, 2nd edn, Dublin 1916

Chadwick, Edwin, *Report on the sanitary condition of the labouring population of Great Britain*, ed. Michael W. Flinn, Edinburgh 1965

Chapman, Carleton B., 'Edward Smith (?1818–1874) physiologist, human ecologist, reformer', *Journal of the History of Medicine and Allied Sciences* xxii (1967), 1–26

Checkland, Sidney, *British public policy 1776–1939*, Cambridge 1983

Chester, Sir Daniel Norman, *The English administrative system, 1780–1870*, London 1981

Clark, George Kitson, 'Statesmen in disguise', *Historical Journal* ii (1959), 19–39

––––––– *The making of Victorian England*, London 1962

Clark, George N., *A history of the Royal College of Physicians of London*, London 1966

Cohen, Emmeline, *The growth of the British civil service, 1780–1939*, London 1941

Cook, Sir Edward, *The life of Florence Nightingale*, London 1913

Creighton, Charles, *A history of epidemics in Britain*, II: *From the extinction of the plague to the present time*, 2nd edn, New York 1965

Cromwell, Valerie, 'Interpretations of nineteenth-century administration: an analysis', *Victorian Studies* ix (1966), 245–54

Crossman, Virginia, *Local government in nineteenth-century Ireland*, Belfast 1994

Crowe, Morgan, 'The origin and development of public health services in Ireland', *The Irish Journal of Medical Science* 6th ser. cclxv (1948), 1–19

Cullen, Michael, *The statistical movement in early Victorian Britain*, New York 1975

Dicey, A. V., *Lectures on the relation between law and public opinion in England during the nineteenth century*, London 1905

Digby, Anne, 'Recent developments in the study of the English poor law', *Local History* xii (1977), 206–11

Donnelly, James S. Jr, 'The administration of relief, 1847–51', in W. E. Vaughn (ed.), *Ireland under the union, I: 1801–70*, Oxford 1989

———— 'Famine and government response, 1845–46', ibid.

Edwards, Ruth Dudley, *An atlas of Irish history*, London 1973

Evans, Eric J. (ed.), *Social policy 1830–1914: individualism, collectivism, and the origins of the welfare state*, Boston 1978

Eyler, John M., 'Mortality statistics and Victorian health policy: program and criticism', *Bulletin of the History of Medicine* l (1976), 335–55

———— *Victorian social medicine: the ideas and methods of William Farr*, Baltimore 1979

Fallon, Martin, *Abraham Colles 1775–1843: surgeon of Ireland*, London 1972

———— (ed.), *The sketches of Erinensis: selections of Irish medical satire, 1824–36*, London 1979

Finer, S. E., *The life and times of Sir Edwin Chadwick*, London 1952

————, 'The transmission of Benthamite ideas 1820–50', in Gillian Sutherland (ed.), *Studies in the growth of nineteenth-century government*, Totowa, NJ 1972

Finnane, Mark, *Insanity and the insane in post-famine Ireland*, London 1981

Fleetwood, John, *A history of medicine in Ireland*, Dublin 1951

Flinn, Michael W., *Public health reform in Britain*, London 1968

———— 'Medical services under the new poor law', in Derek Fraser (ed.), *The new poor law in the nineteenth century*, London 1976, 48–9.

Foster, Roy, *Modern Ireland 1600–1972*, London 1989

Fraser, Derek, *The evolution of the British welfare state: a history of social policy since the Industrial Revolution*, New York 1973

Frazer, William M., *A history of English public health 1834–1939*, London 1950

Freeman, T. W., *Pre-famine Ireland*, Manchester 1957

Froggatt, Peter, 'The response of the medical profession to the great famine', in E. Margaret Crawford (ed.), *Famine: the Irish experience, 900–1900*, Edinburgh 1989

Gash, Norman, *Sir Robert Peel*, Totowa, NJ 1972

Gray, B. Kirkman, *A history of English philanthropy*, London 1905

Hammond, J. L. and Barbara Hammond, *James Stansfeld: a Victorian champion of sex equality*, London 1932

Harley, H. C., 'Sir Henry Acland and his circle', *Oxford Medical School Gazette* xviii (1966), 9–22

Hart, Jenifer, 'Sir John Trevelyan at the Treasury', *English Historical Review* lxxv (1960), 92–111

––––––– 'Nineteenth-century social reform: a Tory interpretation of history', *Past and Present* xxxi (1965), 39–61

Hendriques, Ursula R. Q., *Before the welfare state: social administration in early industrial Britain*, London 1979

Hensey, Brendan, *The health services of Ireland*, 2nd edn, Dublin 1972

Hodgkinson, Ruth G., *The origins of the national health service: the medical services of the new poor law, 1834–71*, London 1967

Holloway, S. W. F., 'Medical education in England, 1830–1858: a sociological analysis', *History* xlix (1964), 299–324

Hoppen, K. Theodore, *Ireland since 1800: conflict and conformity*, New York 1989

Howard-Jones, Norman, 'Cholera therapy in the nineteenth century', *Journal of the History of Medicine* xxvii (1972), 373–95

Hume, L. J., 'Jeremy Bentham and the nineteenth-century revolution in government', *Historical Journal* x (1967), 361–75

––––––– *Bentham and bureaucracy*, Cambridge 1981

Jewson, N. D., 'The disappearance of the sick-man from medical cosmology, 1770–1870', *Sociology* x (1976), 225–44

Keele, Kenneth D., *The evolution of clinical methods in medicine*, Springfield, Ill. 1963

Kinealy, Christine, 'The poor law during the great famine', in Crawford, *Famine*

Lambert, Royston, 'A Victorian national health services: state vaccination, 1855–71', *Historical Journal* v (1962), 1–18

––––––– *Sir John Simon 1816–1904 and English social administration*, London, 1963

Langan, Mary and Bill Schwarz (eds), *Crises in the British state, 1880–1930*, London 1985

Lee, Joseph, *The modernisation of Irish society, 1848–1918*, Dublin 1973

Lewis, Richard A., *Edwin Chadwick and the public health movement, 1832–1854*, London 1952

Liveing, Susan, *A nineteenth-century teacher: John Henry Bridges*, London 1926

Longmate, Norman, *King cholera: the biography of a disease*, London 1966

Loudon, Irvine, *Medical care and the general practitioner, 1750–1850*, Oxford 1986

Lubenow, William C., *The politics of government growth: early Victorian attitudes toward state intervention, 1833–1848*, Hamden, Conn. 1971

Lyons, F. S. L., *Ireland since the famine*, rev. edn, Glasgow 1973

MacArthur, Sir William P., 'Medical history of the famine', in Ruth Dudley Edwards and T. D. Williams (eds) *The great famine: studies in Irish history 1845–52*, Dublin 1956

MacDonagh, Oliver, 'The nineteenth-century revolution in government: a reappraisal', *Historical Journal* i (1958), 52–67

——— *Ireland*, Englewoood Cliffs, NJ 1968

——— *Early Victorian government, 1830–70*, London 1977

McDowell, Robert B., *Public opinion and government policy in Ireland, 1801–46*, London 1952

——— 'Ireland on the eve of the famine', in Dudley Edwards and Williams, *Great famine*

——— *The Irish administration 1801–1914*, London 1964

MacKinnon, Mary, 'English poor law policy and the crusade against outrelief', *Journal of Economic History* xlvii (1987), 603–25

MacLeod, Roy M., 'The frustration of state medicine, 1880–1899', *Medical History* xi (1967), 15–40

——— 'The anatomy of state medicine: concept and application', in F. N. L. Poynter (ed.), *Medicine and science in the 1860s*, London 1968

——— *Treasury control and social administration: a study of establishment growth at the Local Government Board, 1871–1905*, London 1968

——— *Government and expertise: specialists, administrators and professionals, 1860–1914*, Cambridge 1988

McMenemey, William H., *The life and times of Sir Charles Hastings*, Edinburgh–London 1959

Matthew, H. C. G. (ed.), *The Gladstone diaries*, vi–viii, Oxford 1978, 1982

Maxwell, Sir Herbert E., *The life and letters of George William Frederick, fourth earl of Clarendon*, London 1913

Meghen, P. J., 'The development of Irish local government', *Administration* viii (1960), 333–45

——— 'Central–local relationships in Ireland', *Administration* xiii (1965), 107–22

Mitchell, B. R. and Phyllis Deane, *Abstract of British historical statistics*, London 1967

Morley, John, *The life of William Ewart Gladstone*, New York 1903

Newman, Charles, *The evolution of medical education in the nineteenth century*, London 1957

O'Brien, Gerard, 'The new poor law in pre-famine Ireland: a case history', *Irish Economic and Social History* xii (1985), 33–49

O Grada, Cormac, 'Poverty, population and agriculture, 1801–45', in Vaughn, *Ireland under the union, I: 1801–70*

O'Neill, J. E., 'Finding a policy for the sick poor', *Victorian Studies* vii (1964), 264–84

O'Neill, T. P., 'The organisation and administration of relief, 1845–52', in Dudley Edwards and Williams, *Great famine*

——— 'Fever and public health in pre-famine Ireland', *Journal of the Royal Society of Antiquaries of Ireland* ciii (1973), 1–34

O'Tuathaigh, Gearoid, *Ireland before the famine 1798–1848*, Dublin 1972

Owen, David, *English philanthropy 1660–1960*, Cambridge, Mass. 1964

Parris, Henry, 'The nineteenth-century revolution in government: a reappraisal reappraised', *Historical Journal* iii (1960), 17–37

———— *Constitutional bureaucracy: the development of British central adminis-tration since the eighteenth century*, London 1969

Parry, Noel and José Parry, *The rise of the medical profession: a study of collective social mobility*, London 1976

Paz, D. G., 'The limits of bureaucratic autonomy in Victorian adminis-tration', *Historian* xlix (1987), 167–83

Pelling, Margaret, *Cholera, fever and English medicine 1825–1865*, London 1978

Perkin, Harold, *The origins of modern English society*, London 1969

———— 'Individualism versus collectivism in nineteenth-century Britain: a false antithesis', *Journal of British Studies* xvii (1977), 105–18

———— *The rise of professional society*, London 1989

Peterson, M. Jeanne, *The medical profession in mid-Victorian London*, Berkeley–Los Angles 1978

Pickstone, John V., *Medicine and industrial society: a history of hospital develop-ment in Manchester and its region, 1752–1946*, Manchester 1985

Pollak, Kurt and E. Ashworth Underwood, *The healers*, London 1968

Pollitzer, Robert, *Cholera*, Geneva 1959

Porter, Roy, *Disease, medicine and society in England, 1550–1860*, London 1987

Poynter, F. N. L., 'Medical education in England since 1600', in O'Malley, *History of medical education*

Poynter, J. R., *Society and pauperism: English ideas on poor relief, 1795–1834*, London 1969

Prest, John, *Lord John Russell*, Columbia, SC, 1972

Preston-Thomas, Herbert, *The work and play of a government inspector*, Lon-don 1909

Roach, John, *Social reform in England, 1780–1880*, London 1978

Roberts, David, *The Victorian origins of the British welfare state*, New Haven, Conn. 1960

Robins, J. A., 'The Irish hospital: an outline of its origins and development', *Administration* viii (1960), 145–60

Rose, Michael E., *The English poor law 1780–1930*, Newton Abbot 1971

———— 'The crisis of poor relief in England 1860–1890', in W. J. Mommsen (ed.) with Wolfgang Mock, *The emergence of the welfare state in Britain and Germany 1850–1950*, London 1981

Rosen, George, *A history of public health*, New York 1958

Roseveare, Henry, *The Treasury: the evolution of a British institution*, New York 1969

Rowlette, Robert W., *The medical press and circular, 1839–1939: a hundred years in the life of a medical journal*, London 1939

Singer, Charles and E. Ashworth Underwood, *A short history of medicine*, 2nd edn, New York–Oxford 1962

Smith, F. B., *The people's health 1830–1910*, London 1979

———— *Florence Nightingale*, New York 1982

Spinner, Thomas J., *George Joachim Goshen: the transformation of a Victorian liberal*, London 1973

Steele, E. D., *Irish land and British politics*, London 1974

Sutherland, Gillian, 'Recent trends in administrative history', *Victorian Studies* xiii (1970), 408–11

Thomas, Keith, *Religion and the decline of magic*, New York 1971

Tocqueville, Alexis de, *Journeys to England and Ireland*, ed. J. P. Meyer, trans. George Lawrence and J. P. Meyer, New York 1968

Villiers, George, *Vanished Victorian, being the life of George Villiers, fourth earl of Clarendon, 1800–70*, London 1938

Waddington, Ivan, *The medical profession in the industrial revolution*, Dublin 1984

Wain, Harry, *A history of preventive medicine*, Springfield, Ill. 1970

Walsh, James J., *The makers of modern medicine*, New York 1907

Webb, Sidney and Beatrice Webb, *English local government*, vii–x, London 1927–9

Whyte, J. H., *The Independent Irish Party 1850–59*, London 1958

Widdess, J. D. H., *The Royal College of Surgeons in Ireland and its Medical School 1784–1966*, 2nd edn, Edinburgh–London 1967

Winter, James, *Robert Lowe*, Toronto 1976

Wohl, Anthony, *Endangered lives: public health in Victorian Britain*, London 1983

Woodham-Smith, Cecil, *Florence Nightingale, 1820–1910*, London 1951

——— *The great hunger*, London 1962

Woodward, John, *To do the sick no harm: a study of the British voluntary hospital system to 1875*, London–Boston 1974

——— and David Richards (eds), *Health care and popular medicine in nineteenth-century England: essays in the social history of medicine*, New York 1977

Wright, Maurice, *Treasury control of the civil service, 1854–74*, Oxford 1969

Youngson, A. J., *The scientific revolution in Victorian medicine*, New York 1979

Unpublished thesis

Kelly, Patricia, 'From workhouse to hospital: the role of the Irish workhouse in medical relief to 1922', Dublin 1972.

Index